T0210578

Grading Student Midwives' Practice

This book investigates the education and assessment of student midwives in clinical practice, paying particular attention to how their practice is graded.

Chenery-Morris brings primary research, which explores students, mentors, and midwifery lecturers perspectives of practice learning and its assessment, together with the international literature on clinical knowledge, teaching and learning in practice, and assessment of students drawn from a range of healthcare and education professions. Discussing how practice is graded, what constitutes valid practice knowledge, learning in clinical practice, evaluating practice learning, and failing students, this book uses Basil Bernstein's theories to throw light on how we assess and whether we should assess performance in addition to whether a student is competent to practise.

This is an important contribution to the field of midwifery education. It will also be relevant to those with an interest in practice education from a range of healthcare professions.

Sam Chenery-Morris is an Associate Professor in Midwifery and Associate Dean for Learning, Teaching and Student Experience, Head of Nursing and Midwifery, and Lead Midwife for Education at the University of Suffolk. She has worked clinically as a nurse and midwife, as an academic and researcher in her career. Her clinical and pedagogic practice has developed experientially and through academic study over the last 30 years. She has taught midwifery and research modules and been Course Leader for the BSc (Hons) Midwifery [shortened]. She was appointed as an Academic Midwife for the NICE Antenatal Care Clinical Guideline Committee in 2018. This guideline is the largest in the NICE portfolio, and it will shape the care for almost 700,000 pregnant women a year in England and Wales when it is published in 2021.

Routledge Research in Nursing and Midwifery

For more information about this series, please visit: https://www.routledge.com/
Routledge-Research-in-Nursing/book-series/RRIN

Grading Student Midwives' Practice

A Case Study Exploring Relationships, Identity and Authority

Sam Chenery-Morris

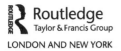
Routledge
Taylor & Francis Group

LONDON AND NEW YORK

First published 2021
by Routledge
2 Park Square, Milton Park, Abingdon, Oxon OX14 4RN

and by Routledge
52 Vanderbilt Avenue, New York, NY 10017

Routledge is an imprint of the Taylor & Francis Group, an informa business

British Library Cataloguing-in-Publication Data
A catalogue record for this book is available from the British Library

Library of Congress Cataloging-in-Publication Data
A catalog record has been requested for this book

ISBN: 978-0-367-43087-0 (hbk)
ISBN: 978-0-367-43088-7 (ebk)

Typeset in Goudy
By Deanta Global Publishing Services, Chennai, India

Contents

Figures

Tables

Preface

This book is the product of more than a decade 'in the field' as a midwifery academic and researcher, supporting students and midwives in clinical practice and teaching in the university setting. Alongside this independent study, Dr Chenery-Morris was a member of a group of midwifery educators, many former or current Lead Midwives for Education, who conducted a five-year, three-phase project on grading practices across the UK. Collectively these endeavours have contributed to the advancements of midwifery education knowledge, specifically related to student's practice learning and assessment. The findings from these studies have been published in various journals, including *Evidence-Based Midwifery*, the *British Journal of Midwifery*, and *Nurse Education in Practice*. Dr Chenery-Morris has also co-authored several midwifery books and is delighted but trepidatious about this, her first solo adventure.

Glossary

Table 0.1 Glossary

Term	Abbreviation (if appropriate)	Definition
Classification	C+/–	A Bernsteinian term referring to the strength of boundary insulation between categories and contexts. Strong classification is explicit differentiation, whereas weak classification is an implicit difference.
Collaborative Learning in Practice	CLiP	New model of practice-based learning where a coach, who is relieved of their clinical responsibilities, facilitates learning for several students (see also PEBLS).
Framing	F+/–	A Bernsteinian term referring to the regulation of the locus of control within categories and contexts. Where framing is strong, the sequencing and pacing of acquisition of knowledge will be controlled by agencies or teachers. Where framing is weak, the student will have greater control.
Invisible pedagogy		A pedagogy invisible to the student which is a manifestation of weak classification and framing rules. Not all students identify with this as learning.
Lead Midwife for Education	LME	A statutory role devised by the Nursing and Midwifery Council. Experienced practising midwife teachers lead on the development, delivery and management of midwifery education programmes within UK universities.
Nursing and Midwifery Council	NMC	The regulatory body in the UK for the professions of nursing and midwifery.
Pedagogic device		The pedagogic device controls who gets what and how, the form and distribution of knowledge.
Pedagogic discourse		Pedagogic discourse refers to the educational transmission code, how students gain access to knowledge.

(Continued)

Term	Abbreviation (if appropriate)	Definition
Pedagogy		A sustained process whereby somebody acquires new forms or develops existing forms of conduct, knowledge, practice and criteria from somebody deemed an appropriate provider and evaluator. Appropriate can be either from the point of view of the acquirer or by some other body or both.
Practice Assessment Document	PAD	A book that students carry to practice, which is used to record mentor signatures when students achieve the NMC and EU competencies. Mentors and students also record the initial, mid-point and endpoint interview and practice grades in the book.
Practice Education Based Learning: Suffolk	PEBLS	New model of practice-based learning where a coach, who is relieved of their clinical responsibilities, facilitates learning for several students (see also CliP).
Practising midwife		Midwife is a protected title for a group of registrants who provide care of women and their families throughout pregnancy, birth and the postnatal period. A distinct profession from nursing. Upon successful completion of an NMC approved course, UK midwives are registered to practice by the NMC.
Practice Assessor		New role introduced in 2018 by the NMC standard for student supervision and assessment.
Practice Supervisor		New role introduced in 2018 by the NMC standard for student supervision and assessment.
Supervisor of Midwives		A role which was statutory in the UK until March 2017. Experienced practising midwives developed and maintained safe practice to ensure public protection by supporting women and midwives.
Visible pedagogy		A pedagogy visible to the student which is a manifestation of strong classification and framing rules.

1 Midwifery, midwifery education and perspectives on grading students' practice

Midwifery is an autonomous profession. Midwives have a unique relationship with a distinct group in society based upon partnership, working with women, their babies and families during pregnancy, birth and the postnatal period. Autonomous midwifery practice enables midwives to fulfil their contract with society by providing up-to-date, evidence-based, high-quality and ethical care for childbearing women and their families (ICM, 2017). Professional autonomy means midwives determine and control the standards for midwifery education, regulation and practice (ICM, 2017).

The word midwife means 'with woman' (Bryar and Sinclair, 2011, p.3), and descriptions of midwives' activities include being with women, being aware of women's feelings, thoughts and experiences by using skills of observation, listening and touch. Being a midwife, one uses the self: a midwife is inextricably linked to the person they are within their relationship with a woman (Bryar and Sinclair, 2011). The ability to be with women and their families is based on personal, empathetic and intuitive qualities supported by knowledge, theory and reflections on practice. Indeed, midwifery has two faces; the public image where midwives deliver woman-centred care and the less visible aspect of midwifery, which is knowledge.

Knowledge comes in many forms: procedural, propositional, practical, personal, tacit, skills and know-how (Eraut, 1994). Understanding midwifery knowledge in its broadest forms will enable a discussion about the relationship between these types of knowledge and their significance for learning and the assessment of students within the profession.

In the UK, the regulatory body for the midwifery profession is the Nursing and Midwifery Council (NMC). The NMC differentiates between the two professions, nursing and midwifery, by producing specific standards for the education of student nurses (NMC, 2010, 2018a) and student midwives (NMC, 2019, 2009). However, the two professions share the standards, or expectations of registrants, that regulate practice and registrant's behaviours (NMC, 2018b).

To become a midwife in the UK prospective students apply to one or more of the 55 universities approved by the NMC to provide midwifery education. Successful applicants undertake the approved midwifery education programme where they acquire the requisite qualification to register with the NMC and practise midwifery. Midwives practice in a variety of settings in the UK, including in the home, the community, hospitals, clinics and birthing units. Students learn to practice by working alongside qualified midwives in addition to undertaking theoretical instruction in the university.

In 2005, and again in 2019, significant changes to the pre-registration midwifery curriculum were considered by the NMC. While the book specifically covers the period between these dates, its relevance to midwifery education continues and, while this is a UK study, the findings could apply to wider audiences. Until March 2017 when it was removed from the statute, the Midwifery Committee advised the NMC on matters affecting midwifery practice, education and supervision. In 2005, a consultation process was undertaken with stakeholder organisations to consider whether midwifery education programmes equipped students to meet the current and future needs of women, babies and families (NMC, 2006). The stakeholders included representatives of user groups, practising midwives, and government and education advisers. The consultation considered:

1. Which competences student midwives should demonstrate,
2. The balance between theory and practice,
3. The minimum academic level for pre-registration midwifery programmes, and
4. Whether practice should be graded and counted towards the degree classification.

Stakeholders had a high level of support for the competences that students would need to demonstrate (between 97 and 100% agreement, ibid.). The competences were physiological, psychological and social knowledge, interpersonal skills, managing emergencies, autonomously supporting normal pregnancy and birth in any setting, and referring women's care when it was recognised to be outside the scope of midwifery practice. Similarly, there was agreement with a flexibility in the division of theory and practice (87%), within the boundary of no less than 40% theory and no more than 60% practice (ibid.). However, concerns were expressed about whether the academic qualification would keep its currency and status with the increased time in practice.

Three-quarters of the panel agreed that practice should be graded (NMC, 2006, p.32) despite reservations that standards to support students' learning and assessment in clinical practice would need to improve. The discussions in the consultation document show that the grading of clinical practice was considered from many perspectives. Grading was considered highly subjective and reliability would be difficult to ensure. The number and differences in midwives' approaches to learning and assessment in clinical practice and the importance of achieving a consistent standard across the UK was considered. As was the possibility of grades skewed towards the higher range. Arguments against grading practice considered that competence has no levels; a student is either competent or not, which equates to safe practitioners. Despite these concerns, the pre-registration standards were published, which included grading students' midwifery practice (NMC, 2009).

The final discussion was whether midwifery education in the UK should become an all graduate profession. There was less support for the move to degree level education (68%) (NMC, 2006). Reticence about raising the academic standard was related to the risk of excluding potential applicants and to the relationship between academic standards and competence in midwifery. However, this too was upheld.

More than a decade later, the standards were revised again after similar consultations (NMC, 2019). This time there was no mandate for the grading of practice, although many midwifery programmes are currently intending to retain this within their curriculum as these are approved from 2020. By 2022 all UK universities will need to adhere to the NMC (2019) standards. The NMC (2019) document was published after my research was concluded; however, the requirements will be referred to and compared to the NMC (2009) standards. This is to maintain the currency of my research to contemporary education discussions and to help inform future iterations of the midwifery curricula development.

In 2009, as a junior member of the midwifery team at Sanderling University (pseudonym), I had limited understanding of the implications of the four changes discussed above and had many questions that informed this research. I was especially interested in how midwives would grade students' practice, how this might affect the student–midwife interactions in the clinical environment and whether the grades would reflect differentiated student performances. If the award of a degree were to retain its academic currency and status, the clinical grade would need to be as exact as possible. However, a qualitative study, published prior to the UK-wide introduction of grading midwifery students' practice, stated that midwives awarded a clinical grade on students' ability to 'do the job' rather than based on assessment criteria (Smith, 2007, p.116). The study of 12 midwives found that some did not feel appropriately qualified to award an academic grade, which caused them stress and anxiety. Participants suggested that students' personalities might influence the grading process, with students who fitted in or those who worked with a similar philosophy to the midwife graded more favourably (Smith, 2007). Devoting time in clinical practice to teaching, supporting and assessing students was also problematic; thus a robust strategy to enable the assessment and grading of clinical practice at degree level was recommended (Smith, 2007).

The importance of a consistent standard across the UK and a suitable period to allow grading of clinical competence to be developed were documented by the stakeholders of the consultation (NMC, 2006). The Midwifery Committee agreed that further work would be done in relation to how grading clinical practice via education providers would be implemented (NMC, 2006). However, no further updates were posted on the website as agreed. The grading of practice workshops were delivered nationally, but individual universities were responsible for developing local grading tools. Some universities worked together in regions to develop grading tools, but most worked independently.

The significance of assessing students' practice cannot be overstated. The NMC's primary function is to protect the public. The standards for pre-registration midwifery education state what universities and practice must do to ensure that students, after a period of education, are safe to practice (NMC, 2009, 2019). The competencies and types of assessments are clearly stated, and quality assured to ensure public protection. However, there has been research in nursing and midwifery, suggesting that mentors 'fail to fail' (Duffy, 2004; Fraser, 1988).

The term mentor was specific to this period (beginning in 2006 until 2020) and referred to a midwife (or nurse) who had undertaken an approved NMC qualification to teach and assess students in clinical practice. Despite the qualification, the 'failure to fail' literature suggests that some students became registered nurses or midwives without the requisite attitude, knowledge or skills because the staff assessing their practice had not failed the student in their practice assessments. The introduction of grading midwifery students' clinical practice may have been suggested as a remedy to the 'failure to fail' phenomenon. However, no rationale for its introduction was stated at the time.

Given the lack of midwifery research on grading clinical practice, it seemed pertinent to study issues around grading practice. Therefore, this chapter first reports on a comprehensive review of the literature, considering:

1. How practice is assessed,
2. By whom,
3. The typical practice grades from a range of health professions, and
4. Issues with grading practice before outlining the research questions to be addressed in this book.

1.1 The literature review

As is typical with many forms of research, I started with a review of the available literature to understand the field, how others had researched the topic and to identify a potential gap in the research (Ridley, 2008; Hart, 1988). This enabled me to understand how I would plan and conduct research on grading clinical practice. Subsequently, I formulated research questions and utilised a suitable research design to answer these. The methodical search of the literature was undertaken at the beginning of the research project in 2009 and a further search in December 2016 using databases: CINHAL via EBSCOhost, Health and Medicine Proquest, Medline and Google Scholar (Appendix 1). The combination of 'practice' and 'grade' were used as keywords to search the databases. The synonyms appraise, evaluate, performance and competence were also used initially to source the literature; however, while this increased the number of potential sources, it did not increase the specificity of the search.

Several studies have researched simulation techniques, and used virtual patients or portfolios as mechanisms to grade clinical practice. These were excluded as I wanted research that assessed clinical practice in its authentic setting rather than a proxy. Opinion papers and those not concerning grading in healthcare clinical settings were excluded. After reading the title and abstract of all potential papers, 34 research papers were included in my review. The review includes a literature review (n=1), a large-scale action research project (n=1), surveys (n=13), audits or analyses of practice grades, (n=13) and qualitative studies (n=6).

At the start of my research, the most comprehensive and often cited reports by Gray and Donaldson (2009a, 2009b) were useful sources of information. The reports, published in two volumes, were commissioned by NHS Education for Scotland in response to the NMC's decision to grade student midwives' practice (Gray and Donaldson, 2009a, 2009b). A further publication using the same literature was produced three years later (Donaldson and Gray, 2012). The authors systematically searched health education literature finding 119 studies from a range of professional groups where practice was graded. One limitation of their literature review is that some papers were included that were not based on empirical data. The authors acknowledge this, having included 28 articles based on description or opinion. The remaining literature included quantitative studies (n=66), literature reviews (n=19) or qualitative research (n=6).

While the research is cited often, like all studies, it has limitations. The literature review process in the earlier reports (Gray and Donaldson, 2009a, 2009b) clearly stated the keywords and databases used, but the search strategy was not presented, so the study could not be replicated. However, this was apparent in the later publication (Donaldson and Gray, 2012). In this publication, it is stated that 28 of the 119 studies were found from hand searching or back chaining through journals. Thus a high proportion of papers were not found in the systematic phase of the search. Additionally, I question the inclusion of two of the qualitative studies as they are not specifically about grading practice but mentorship instead. This slightly undermines the objectivity of their review. Although they did not focus solely on empirical studies, it is still comprehensive, and the authors managed to source a greater number of publications than my later search.

The Gray and Donaldson reports (2009a, 2009b) state the reasons for and against the grading of clinical practice, as well as the tensions with this form of assessment. They compared 16 grading tools from the literature published between 1999–2009. The grading tools were considered under-developed in terms of their effectiveness, usefulness, reliability and validity (Gray and Donaldson, 2009a, p.4). Grade inflation was noted and assigned to four influences:

1. The student
2. The assessor
3. The student–assessor relationship
4. The grading tools

Their recommendations, if grading practice was adopted, was for the development and testing of rubrics, multiple methods of assessment, training of assessors and evaluation of the grading processes. Thus, at the time grading of practice was introduced to midwifery education, there was little sound evidence to suggest it would be beneficial.

The empirical evidence from my literature search incorporates the tensions noted above but also considers:

1. How practice is assessed
2. The practice grades
3. Relationships in clinical practice

Each of these will be considered in turn, especially in relation to the reliability and validity of graded practice assessments.

1.1.1 *How is practice graded?*

Fifteen of the reviewed papers stated how practice was assessed or graded (Table 1.1). The definition of 'grade' used, in relation to my work and the literature, was a mark indicating the quality of a student's practice. Assessment, alternatively, was used to evaluate, judge or appraise the quality of students' practice performance. There seemed to be a shared understanding of how practice was graded or assessed. The commonalities most often cited across the professions were with observation, skills testing, oral exams and student self-assessment.

Table 1.1 is presented in five categories. I grouped the method of assessment into similar approaches based on the technique used to assess the students' practice. The first is observation. An assessor could observe or watch a student taking a client's history or performing skills and make a decision based on the students' performance. The underlying reasons for why they asked questions, or not, and their knowledge would not necessarily be known, but the performance could be examined.

Oral assessments, alternatively, were used for students to articulate their decision making processes and application of these to care. Oral assessment could be part of a history taking observation, but this was not always explicitly stated, therefore, I concluded, this was a separate, second form of assessment. There was often an explicit rationale, such as to foreground knowledge, for this method. Student self-assessment is the third category on its own. It was rarely used as a sole method of assessment. Often it was rationalised as a strategy to increase students' professional development.

The fourth category, exams and portfolios, were grouped together as they represented written work, rather than practical skills. Students may write about their performance, but the relationship between their essay and practice is unknown. Lastly, conference presentations were removed from the actual clinical environment and considered a separate form of assessment. The table shows there are many methods used to assess students' practice, with some preferred methods in each profession. The rationale and limitation of each method need to be considered when developing curricula to determine the best approach and method that measures the skills being assessed.

Several perspectives and approaches have been used to research grading practices in the healthcare professions and the body of evidence is derived from this

Table 1.1 Methods used to grade or assess practice from the reviewed literature

Method	Professions	References
Observation	Nursing, physiotherapy, midwifery, medicine	Clouder and Toms, 2008; Meldrum et al., 2008; Dalton et al., 2009; Oermann et al., 2009; Hatfield and Lovegrove, 2012; Plakht et al., 2013; Paskausky and Simonelli, 2014; Murphy et al., 2014; Fisher et al., 2017; Imanipour and Jalili, 2016; Lawson et al., 2016.
Skills testing	Nursing, medicine, midwifery	Pulito et al., 2007; Oermann et al., 2009; Imanipour and Jalili, 2016.
Physical exam	Medicine, nursing	Eggleton et al., 2016; Imanipour and Jalili, 2016.
History taking	Medicine, nursing	Eggleton et al., 2016; Imanipour and Jalili, 2016.
Supervised interviews	Medicine	Briscoe et al., 2006.
Case presentation	Medicine, nursing	Briscoe et al., 2006; Imanipour and Jalili, 2016.
Measurement of humanistic qualities	Medicine, nursing	Eggleton et al., 2016; Imanipour and Jalili, 2016.
Diagnostic ability	Medicine	Pulito et al., 2007.
Oral examinations	Physiotherapy, medicine, nursing, midwifery	Briscoe et al., 2006; Pulito et al., 2007; Clouder and Toms, 2008; Reubenson et al., 2012; Fisher et al., 2017; Imanipour and Jalili, 2016.
Self-assessment	Nursing	Oermann et al., 2009; Hatfield and Lovegrove, 2012; Plakht et al., 2013.
Final exams	Medicine, nursing	Briscoe et al., 2006; Paskausky and Simonelli, 2014.
Written assignments	Nursing, medicine	Oermann et al., 2009; Briscoe et al., 2006.
Portfolio	Midwifery	Fisher et al., 2017.
Conference presentations	Nursing	Oermann et al., 2009.

eclectic mix. Most of the studies were local evaluations of grading tools (Clouder and Toms, 2008; Meldrum et al., 2008; Hatfield and Lovegrove, 2012; Plakht et al., 2013; Murphy et al., 2014; Eggleton et al., 2016; Imanipour and Jalili, 2016), but there were a few national surveys of grading practices in nursing, midwifery and medicine (Oermann et al., 2009; Fisher et al., 2017; Lawson et al., 2016). One action research study developed a national grading tool for physiotherapy (Dalton et al., 2009). Studies also focussed on the relationship between performance criteria (Pulito et al., 2007), or exam and practice grades (Paskausky and Simonelli, 2014), the nature of graded assessments (Briscoe et al., 2006) and agreement between examiners (Meldrum et al., 2008; Dalton et al., 2009; Reubenson et al., 2012; Eggleton et al., 2016).

The weight of the evidence is limited by the size, generalisability and transferability of some of the studies. For instance, the quantitative studies tended to be small scale local surveys, as small as one student and seven examiners (Reubenson et al., 2012). Even the larger national surveys had methodological issues. For instance, Oermann et al. (2009) emailed 21,719 members of a nursing network asking for full- or part-time faculty to respond. The sample of respondents who were eligible was not known, those who responded were self-selected, and the numbers from each university were not stated. The representativeness of the sample was unknown, and therefore the generalisability of the findings is compromised. One of the most rigorous studies, was the largescale, two phase action research project of over a thousand participants from multiple universities across New Zealand and Australia which developed a national grading tool for physiotherapy (Dalton et al., 2009). However, once the grading tool was developed, there was only a limited evaluation of it by students. Thus, the evidence across the studies of how best to grade practice is not robust.

I questioned whether all the forms of assessment presented in Table 1.1 could measure practice. To consider this point Miller's pyramid (1990) is used to show the distinct types of practice knowledge related to the assessment methods. Miller's pyramid traditionally illustrates four stages of knowledge, which can be separated into two types; those that can be assessed by traditional methods such as exams and written tests and those that measure the application of knowledge in the workplace. The first two are typically cognitive measures; knows and knows how. Whereas, the upper levels are behavioural or practical; shows and does.

Behaviours or practice knowledge can be observed as in 'observation' or specifically in activities such as a 'physical exam' (as seen in Table 1.1). However, 'knowing' and 'knowing how', it can be argued, do not necessarily equate to 'showing how' or 'doing'. Clouder and Toms (2008) argue that 'doing' and appearing competent can mask limited understanding and practice assessments should have both observation and a rationale (theoretical underpinnings) for the action.

One interpretation of Miller's pyramid is that knowledge is the foundation on which practice is built. However, it could be argued that knowledge and competence are lower-order skills than performance and action. Whether one can perform without some knowledge can be debated, but in the clinical environment the third and fourth levels are typically assessed (Clouder and Toms, 2008). From this pyramid, one can see how the emphasis of assessment of competence and/or performance shifts the balance of power in the direction of practice away from theory (Norris, 1991). The implication here could be that action is more important than the underpinning knowledge, especially if observation is used as a sole method to grade practice. I will come back to this point in the book, because all professions have a specific body of knowledge that they profess. Without this specific knowledge the care they provide could be any generic healthcare rather

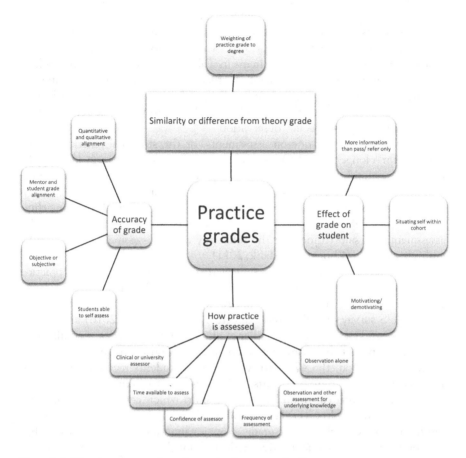

Figure 1.1 Visual representation of quantitative survey findings.

than, in the case of this research, explicitly midwifery care. If the midwifery profession values the knowledge that makes it unique, it needs to ensure it teaches
and assesses students in that discipline. Action alone is insufficient to embody
midwifery practice; the midwife needs the requisite underpinning knowledge to
offer women choices and discussion to fully consent to their care.

Each method of assessment is now considered to examine the strength of evidence from the literature.

1.1.2 Observation of practice

The four national studies that reported on practice assessment types all used
observation as a method to grade practice (Dalton et al., 2009; Oermann et al.,
2009; Fisher et al., 2017; Lawson et al., 2016). The studies represent different

professions and countries, including the UK, USA, New Zealand and Australia. Despite being the most often used method, for example, 93% (n=1289) of nursing programmes in the US (Oermann et al., 2009), observation was not a universally described method and observation of 'what' was not always explicitly stated. One could assume the first seven items in Table 1.1 under observation include a stated activity rather than general observation. In nursing and medicine, for instance, students were observed undertaking a physical exam or patient history (Eggleton et al., 2016; Imanipour and Jalili, 2016); however, these activities may also be part of the less specific 'observation'.

Observations can be one-off assessments, or the students' practice can be observed for a longer period. One-off assessments are sometimes considered to be high stakes, snapshot assessments as a competence or grade may be determined by one or a few discrete assessment points (Bhugra and Malik, 2011). How a student behaves on the given day may not reflect how they usually perform; thus, a student may fail who would usually pass and vice versa. More frequent one-off assessments are said to increase the reliability of the assessment, especially by multiple assessors (Bhugra and Malik, 2011).

Medical students tended to be subject to frequent observations of practice in the form of daily shift scorecards (Weaver et al., 2007; Lurie and Mooney, 2010; Hiller et al., 2016; Lawson et al., 2016). However, two of the studies, the national US survey of 100 medical directors (Lawson et al., 2016) and a local study of 47 student evaluations (Hiller et al., 2016), noted widespread difficulty with compliance of shift card scores. These were often late or not returned. In a ten-month period, the 47 fourth-year medical students received on average 11 clinical evaluations from 12 shifts (Hiller et al., 2016). Some report cards were not completed until two months after the shift, which could compromise the quality of the data. However, Hiller et al. (2016) found no association between the timing of feedback and the grade. A major limitation of their study is that they only analysed the quantitative grade and not the qualitative comments on the reports. Anecdotally they observed that the reports completed sooner tended to have a greater quantity and more specific feedback to the students (Hiller et al., 2016) but as these comments were not part of the research this form of potentially rich data was not analysed. Lawson et al.'s (2016) national study corroborated Hiller et al.'s (2016) findings about low return rates and lengthy delays before the completion of shift cards, for these reasons they questioned the quality of this method of assessment.

In Fisher et al.'s (2017) survey of UK grading practices, the frequency of midwifery students' practice assessments ranged from once or twice per year to a variety throughout the year. The grades may have been collected at these times, but the observation of clinical practice was based on a longer period of assessment; regulated by the NMC (2009, 2008). Regular or continuous assessment is said to provide a greater opportunity for feedback to students and more sampling of students' practice for assessors (Bhugra and Malik, 2011). It has been considered a more valid, reliable and realistic practice assessment method. However, Girot (1993) challenged this notion, saying that continuous assessment is 'no assessment at all' as assessors in clinical practice have limited time to supervise or give the necessary feedback to students (Girot, 1993). More than 20 years later it is noted, albeit in small local surveys, that students still want to spend more time with their assessors observing their practice (Hanley and Higgins, 2005) and being available for quality feedback is also still problematic (Susmarini and Hayati, 2011). Thus the observation of a longer period of practice is not without its limitations.

Five studies explored the reliability of observation of practice between examiners (Pulito et al., 2007; Meldrum et al., 2008; Dalton et al., 2009; Reubenson et al., 2012; Eggleton et al., 2016). Four of the studies said the assessments were reliable or demonstrated consistency between examiners; only one said the opposite (Pulito et al., 2007). However, I argue that two of the studies did not prove inter-rater reliability. Both used videos of student performances to measure inter-rater reliability (Reubenson et al., 2012; Eggleton et al., 2016). In Reubenson et al. (2012), there was one physiotherapy student and seven examiners. Whereas, Eggleton et al. (2016) had three staged performances representing fail (grade 1) a borderline pass (grade 2), pass (grade 3) or distinction (grade 4) and 100 General Practioner assessors. Both studies noted a range of marks awarded from 1–3 or 1–4 (Eggleton et al., 2016) and 40–70% (Reubenson et al., 2012) with a pass mark of 50%. Thus both studies had examiners awarding pass and fail grades for the same student performance. These small scale studies show major discrepancies in differentiating student performances if the examiners do not agree on the minimum threshold that a student has to achieve to pass. The broad range of performances, from fail to distinction and across the 40–70 percentage range, further undermines the reliability of this form of assessment.

While I considered Dalton et al.'s (2009) study to be rigorous in developing a national grading tool, when assessing the inter-rater reliability of the tool only 30 pairs of students and assessors over a 4–6-week placement were measured. The findings documented a 68% confidence interval that scores were accurate to within plus or minus two points, although they do not explain the significance of the points (Dalton et al., 2009). This means that 32% of assessments were not accurate or not within the pre-specified accuracy measure. A larger physiotherapy study performed over five placements of 4–6 weeks, with 86 paired assessment forms, one graded by an educator, the other by tutors, also noted consistency in 74% of the assessments (Meldrum et al., 2008). No students failed this assignment, so all assessors agreed pass grades; however, there were differences between student grades, most often between the higher grade boundaries, and 26% were not consistent. Meldrum et al. (2008) documented, due to confidentiality, they were unable to say how many students the forms measured and stated some students may have been assessed three times by different assessor pairs. Thus, fewer than 86 students may have been observed.

Only one study in the review recorded low inter-reliability (Pulito et al., 2007). The study of 211 student grades by two or three assessors resulted in 585 evaluations. Pulito et al. found that the judgement of one doctor did not correlate highly with the perceptions of another. They found the assessors formed an overall impression of the student, often based on personal qualities such as professionalism or interpersonal skills rather than diagnostic skills (Pulito et al., 2007). To me this is part of the reason why reliability between assessors is compromised.

Professionalism and interpersonal skills are subjective measures and therefore there will be differences between assessors' expectations and whether a student can meet these. While not stated, it may explain why some students passed with high grades and others were failed in the Eggleton et al. (2016) and Reubenson et al. (2012) studies. Even where consistency is noted above, albeit on exceedingly small samples, a quarter of the cases revealed no consistency between assessors (Meldrum et al., 2008; Dalton et al., 2009).

Amicucci (2012) questioned the subjective nature of practice grades in a phenomenological study of face-to-face interviews with 11 faculty members with master's degrees. The participants considered classroom grades more objective than practice grades. The friends and family test, which asks whether the assessor would want this student caring for them, was used. A problem with this test is the assumption that all the patients would have the same values and beliefs and therefore want the same care as the assessors. It might also explain why in a further small scale qualitative study of 11 students, that some commented on 'very different assessments from different assessors' (Hanley and Higgins, 2005, p.280). As each assessor-student relationship is unique, there may be limited consistency.

In summary, while observation is an often-used method to assess practice, there are multiple issues in terms of the evidence base for frequency, compliance, reliability and the subjective nature of the grading process. There is conflicting evidence of consistency between assessors; however, most of the research used small samples and evaluated local practices, so the strength of the evidence for the use of observation as a valid method of assessment is limited. Perhaps due to these limitations, many programmes used two or more methods of assessment (as seen in Table 1.1).

1.1.3 Other methods to assess practice; incorporating theoretical knowledge

While observation enables the observer to see what the student is doing, the rationale for their action is not visible. Thus, three of the included studies researched ways to deliberately incorporate students' knowledge base into the practice assessment by having an oral assessment as well as direct observation (Pulito et al., 2007; Clouder and Toms, 2008; Imanipour and Jalili, 2016). Oral presentations, rather than exams, were considered an accurate way to assess medical students practice in an analysis of faculty assigned grades (Pulito et al., 2007). In logistic regression tests, the oral exam was predictive of the overall student grade ($p=<0.001$) with 83% accuracy. A strength of this study is that it used inferential statistics and quantified statistical significance with its findings. However, their conclusion was that the oral presentation had a limited increase in the overall accuracy of grades and was as reliable as measuring professionalism, clinical skills and patient management, presumably by observation (Pulito et al., 2007).

The other two studies looked specifically at oral exams and participants' experiences (Clouder and Toms, 2008; Imanipour and Jalili, 2016). Both studies examined whether observation and other methods were necessary from student and assessors' perspectives. The oral exam was said to have a high educational impact by the students and assessors alike; this meant the assessment was considered objective, clear and feasible with a positive impact on learning (Clouder and Toms, 2008; Imanipour and Jalili, 2016). Clouder and Toms' (2008) qualitative study was explicit in the number and types of participants (n=55) including students, clinical educators and university tutors with varying levels of experience and both genders. Rigour was maintained through the qualitative concept of trustworthiness, participant validation and triangulation (Clouder and Toms, 2008). Participants considered both assessment types, direct observation and the oral exam necessary for practice but for distinct reasons.

The students considered the oral assessment necessary to articulate the assessment of the client and encouraged them to learn (Clouder and Toms, 2008). Whereas, educators found the distance between the students and themselves enabled the assessment to be more objective (ibid.). The oral exam was thought to enable better differentiation between student performances. Assessors disclosed they were sometimes surprised by the student oral performances as they did not always match their expectations, with some students who were believed to be excellent not performing well and vice versa (Clouder and Toms, 2008). Educators said the depth of knowledge students expressed was inspiring and illuminating, and it aided students in their professional development (Clouder and Toms, 2008). A limitation the authors acknowledged was that the context of learning was not evaluated as their study focussed on the assessment of learning.

Four methods of assessment, including an oral exam, were introduced and evaluated positively in nursing in Japan (Imanipour and Jalili, 2016). All four assessments, direct observation, a specific rating score, oral examination and professional behaviours were considered necessary to assess practice. The oral exam was considered by experts in the field to have a higher content validity index, i.e. its relevancy, clarity and simplicity, than direct observation of practice, but observation had a higher content validity ratio, i.e. it was necessary. The number and where the experts were drawn from is not stated. However, both methods were considered reliable using Cronbach's alpha coefficient (Imanipour and Jalili, 2016). Students (n=38) and instructors (n=8) were surveyed about the new tools and agreed that the direct observation and oral exam had a positive impact on learning (87% instructors and 89% students) (Imanipour and Jalili, 2016).

Other methods were also used, seemingly less frequently, to assess practice (Table 1.1) such as final examinations (Briscoe et al., 2006; Paskausky and Simonelli, 2014), written assignments (Oermann et al., 2009) and portfolios (Fisher et al., 2017). Whether these can be considered applied theoretical assessments, or stand alone, as the underpinning knowledge for practice can be debated. However, these assessments are outside the remit of this work for the reasons stated earlier, that I wanted to study authentic clinical assessments.

1.2 Who grades practice?

Differences were noted in who completed the practice assessments. In nursing and midwifery in the UK, registrants working in clinical practice typically assessed students (Hanley and Higgins, 2005; Hatfield and Lovegrove, 2012; Fisher et al., 2017). This was due to UK regulation from the NMC that stated who was able to assess nursing and midwifery students (NMC, 2008). In the United States, nursing faculty, those working in universities, visited students in practice to assign a clinical grade (Scanlan and Care, 2004; Walsh and Seldomridge, 2005; Seldomridge and Walsh, 2006; Pulito et al., 2007; Paskausky and Simonelli, 2014). One might assume university staff would be familiar with assigning grades for theory and therefore confident assigning practice grades. However, in the literature, a key theme was that some assessors lacked confidence in grading students' practice, regardless of whether the assessor was based in the university or clinical environment.

In the UK national survey of Lead Midwives for Education, participants asserted that clinicians were confident to award practice grades, and the confidence increased over time (Fisher et al., 2017). These findings need to be considered with caution, as clinicians themselves were not surveyed. However, the findings from Fisher et al.'s (2017) study are similar to findings by Heaslip and Scammell (2012) where clinicians' views were sought. In Heaslip and Scammell's (2012) survey, 64.3% (n=72) of the 112 nursing mentors expressed confidence in grading practice; only 10% stated that they were not confident. When a further question regarding confidence to fail a student was asked, 59.5% (n=67) indicated that they were confident; however, 17.8% (n=5) reported a lack of confidence (Heaslip and Scammell, 2012, p.99). Whether this is statistically significant or not is not known because the study only reports descriptive statistics. Nevertheless, it is significant to note that not all mentors were confident to grade or fail students' practice, despite having the requisite qualification to gain mentor status.

A similar finding, of a lack of confidence, stress and anxiety about the grading process, was described in a small qualitative study (Smith, 2007). Smith (2007) interviewed 12 midwifery mentors from a population of 72. While 30 mentors agreed to take part, Smith stratified the respondents in terms of academic backgrounds to encompass a random sample. This adds to the credibility of the research because the sample was as diverse as possible. The author noted that a lack of experience in grading students' practice may have contributed to the mentor's lack of confidence. She suggested that over time, as grading became more established, this might improve (Smith, 2007). This belief was corroborated by the Fisher et al. (2017) study.

Greater confidence was expressed in the Docherty and Dieckmann (2015) cross-sectional descriptive survey of 84 medical faculties across 14 separate educational settings who awarded clinical grades. They found that 88% of doctors were confident to determine grades. However, the low survey response rate of 33% could be attributed to a bias towards only the most confident replying. It is concerning that 66% of respondents said they worked with students who should not have passed and 72% admitted giving students grades that afforded the benefit of the doubt. These findings reveal a contradiction in respondents' responses. Despite confidence to determine grades, there was uncertainty as to whether the students should be awarded the grades they received. If an assessor is confident, there should be no need to give the student the benefit of the doubt (Docherty and Dieckmann, 2015). It also raises the question of the reliability of the practice grade if so many assessors have worked with students whose practice may not meet the minimum standard.

There was low confidence that faculty could discriminate appropriately between student performances in a national survey of doctors (Briscoe et al., 2006). While half of the 85 respondents thought they 'frequently' could, 41.7% felt they did so 'occasionally' (Briscoe et al., 2006). Therefore, the reliability of the assessment is again questioned. The 'failure to fail' literature with competence or graded assessments is prolific and will be considered later in the book in relation to midwifery students whose practice is not considered adequate (Duffy, 2004; McGregor, 2007; Luhanga et al., 2008; Larocque and Luhanga, 2013; Hunt et al., 2016; Scalan and Chernomas, 2016). The key conclusion of much of the literature from practice assessors was that faculty or clinical mentors, wanted more support to grade students' practice (Briscoe et al., 2006; Smith, 2007; Heaslip and Scammell, 2012).

1.2.1 Student self-assessment

In some of the studies, nursing students self-assessed their practice (Table 1.1). It is paradoxical that research questioned the appropriateness of this form of assessment and its accuracy when the sections above have questioned these aspects when qualified staff grade practice. The method, accuracy and confidence of the assessor all affected the assessment of students' practice, so student self-assessment is likely to be equally problematic. None of the studies used student self-assessment as a sole method to grade practice, probably because students on nursing programmes would need to be assessed by qualified staff to be eligible to enter the professional register. However, reflective practice and self-assessment of performance is a key skill in many professions so it would seem appropriate this form of assessment is used alongside other methods (Oermann et al., 2009).

In Hatfield and Lovegrove's (2012) survey, only 48% of the 65 assessors (n=31) considered that students could self-assess their performance. Half the assessors (n=33) thought students could not, leaving one assessor with no opinion (Hatfield and Lovegrove, 2012). It should be noted that the response rate to this survey was low (38%). Nonetheless, 23% of assessors (n=15) thought students assessed their performance too low, with 9% (n=6) stating that students inflated their grades. Participants suggested that students inflated their grade because they had limited insight into their practice. There was also the potential that the assessor would agree with the elevated grade. The literature presented above identified some mentors who had low confidence in grade practice; therefore, a confident student may be able to influence their grade. This is a concern for students on professional courses because an assessment should be reliable.

The accuracy of 124 student nursing practice grades and student self-assessment was surveyed by Plakht et al. (2013). A strength of this survey is the use of inferential statistics to show that 60% of student grades were considered accurate when compared to their assessors' grade. A quarter of students self-assessed their performance as lower and 15% were higher than their mentor's grade (Plakht et al., 2013). When compared to Hatfield and Lovegrove's (2012) data, a similar percentage of students had lower grades (23% compared to 25%). However, more students over-estimated their performance than the mentors thought (9% compared to 15%). As the reliability of the practice grade is in question, it would seem student self-assessment is no more or less accurate than assessors' grades.

The quality of the feedback from the mentor was considered important in enabling students to self-assess (Plakht et al., 2013). High-quality negative feedback enabled students to align their scores to the mentors more than high-quality positive feedback. Positive feedback led to an over estimation of student performance, especially if the student received a 'very high' evaluation (Plakht et al., 2013). Next in this chapter, the practice grades are compared to show that most students receive 'very high' evaluations for practice. This could limit students' ability for accurate self-assessment and reflection. The implication of Plakht et al.'s (2013) research is that assessors are impeding students' self-evaluation by focusing on positive feedback rather than on areas for development. Potential reasons for this will also be considered.

1.3 The practice grades

There were 14 studies that stated or analysed the practice grades, with a variety of grade types.

Collectively Table 1.2 proves that practice grades tend to be clustered towards the higher end of the grade ranges regardless of the grading type; letter, mean or descriptor. It appears that some phenomenon could be attributable to the higher practice grades. It may be that practice is harder to assess, that the assessment needs to combine multiple parts to be more reliable, that the assessment, often based on observation, is not capable of stratifying students or that the relationship between students and assessors affects the grades. Nonetheless, the implication of this on healthcare students' degree classifications is not negligible. It will depend on the balance between theory and practice and the contribution each has on the degree classification. The currency and status of the academic award could be eroded if more credits are derived from the practice assessments where students are typically awarded higher grades.

The largest retrospective study of 4500 student nurses' practice grades, collected over 25 years in Canada, found that 90% of grades were B+ and above, and 60% of grades A or A+ (Scanlan and Care, 2004). In the final practicum, 80% of the clinical grades were A or A+, and only 3% of students received a B or lower (Scanlan and Care, 2004). A similar pattern of high grades with year-on-year increases was found in the UK in 1057 occupational therapy students'

Table 1.2 Practice grades

Grading type	Grade/mean	Number of grading episodes	Author
Mean	93%	124	Plakht et al., 2013,
	4.1/5 (range 2.3–5) SD 0.62 (82% range 69–100%)	547	Hiller et al., 2016,
	3.3–3.72/4 (range 82–93%)	184	Walsh and Seldomridge, 2005,
	84% in the older tool (range 69–99%) to 78% in the newer tool (range 62–92%)	71	Murphy et al., 2014, the same study awarded grades in two ways.
Descriptor	Excellent (41%), good (52%), adequate (7%), not adequate (Combined good and excellent = 93% of students)	71	Murphy et al., 2014.
Range	60–72%	1057	Roden, 2016,
	40–70%	7	Reubenson et al., 2012,
	5.5–8/9 (61–89%)	100	Eggleton et al., 2016,
	80–95%	281	Paskausky and Simonelli, 2014.
Letter	A or B (combined = 95% of grades)	204	Seldomridge and Walsh, 2006,
	68% A; 32% B (combined = 100% of grades)	585	Pulito et al., 2007,
	90% higher than B+	281	Paskausky and Simonelli, 2014,
	A or A+ 80% in the last practicum	4500	Scanlan and Care, 2004.
Honours/ pass/ fail	22% honours, 49% strong pass, 28% pass, 0 fail. Upper 5% = 9.8% upper 25% = 41.2% expected = 46% below = 2.8% far below 0	3369	Weaver et al., 2007.
Not stated but high	5% fell outside the cluster but no value is given meaning 95% similar	38	Edwards, 2012.

grades over five years (Roden, 2016). The second- and third-year practice grades were considered statistically significant (Roden, 2016). In the final-year student practice grades ranged from 67–72% on a 48-item criterion-referenced practice report. Both studies showed that grades for practice increased each year despite the higher level required (Scanlan and Care, 2004; Roden, 2016).

In a before and after study of 3349 medical student evaluations, Weaver et al. (2007) altered the shift card from four grade descriptors (honours, high pass, pass and fail) to five (upper 5%, upper 25%, expected level, below expected level and far below). Before the change (n=1612 evaluations), 22.6% of the student evaluations were at the honours level, 49% high pass and 28.4% pass, with no fail grades. After the change (n=1737 evaluations), fewer students received the highest grades, with 9.8% awarded upper 5% and 41.2% graded upper 25% (Weaver et al., 2007). Almost half the students were deemed to be at the expected level (46%), and while no students were far below the expected level, a few (2.8%) were deemed to be below expectations (Weaver et al., 2007). The more explicit criteria were found to reduce the number of very high practice grades. Although interestingly, 51% of student evaluations were still noted to be in the upper quarter.

While all three studies (Scanlan and Care, 2004; Weaver et al., 2007; Roden, 2016) were undertaken in a single university, the size of the data sets, number of cohorts examined and similarity with other research (Table 1.2) mean the strength of evidence for high practice grades is strong. It is also worth acknowledging that the grades were awarded by a variety of health professionals, those working in clinical practice and in universities, yet they were nearly all at the higher end of the grade spectrum.

When grading students' practice became mandatory in the UK, 50% of the 40 Lead Midwives for Education who replied (73% response rate) to a national survey reported that student grade profiles had increased (Fisher et al., 2017). This is no doubt due to the inclusion of practice grades to the overall degree classification. No lead midwives reported lower practice grades. Some were unable to tell whether grading practice influenced the grades. They had either been grading students' practice for longer than ten years or had only recently introduced it (Fisher et al., 2017). The lead midwives said that where grading had been common practice for more than ten years, the grades lowered over time as mentors became more confident and used the full spectrum of grades (Fisher et al., 2017), although no evidence for this was presented.

Many of the studies showed narrow grade ranges, particularly Walsh and Seldomridge (2005), Edwards (2012) and Paskausky and Simonelli (2014). While Edwards (2012) attributed this phenomenon to consistency between assessors, Walsh and Seldomridge (2005) suggested that the grading criteria were too broad and that the lack of specificity in differentiating between grades was part of the problem. They also said that some aspects of clinical practice are harder to measure and compared psychomotor skills with clinical interactions, suggesting the former is more straightforward to assess than the latter (Walsh and Seldomridge, 2005). As clinical performance is made up of many episodes of clinical interactions, the evidence suggests the assignation of the practice grade is imprecise.

1.3.1 Grade inflation

I questioned whether the high practice grades represented grade inflation. Grade inflation in the literature was identified in four forms.

1. An individual student received a higher grade than their performance warranted
2. Trends over time as grades for successive cohorts increase
3. The difference between theory and practice grades
4. The contribution of practice grades to the overall degree

Two national surveys of medical education confirmed students often received grades higher than their practice called for (Briscoe et al., 2006; Fazio et al., 2013), with a worrying number of participants disclosing that students were passed when they did not meet the acceptable level. When a sample of 69 clinical directors from the 143 medical schools in the US and Canada were surveyed (Fazio et al., 2013) most respondents, 55% (n=38), thought that grade inflation existed although many (41%) thought that it was more problematic at a school other than their own; 38% of participants agreed that students had passed who should not have. The study had a reasonable response rate of 48%. This is supported by another national survey with a slightly better response rate (66%) of 85 medical directors (Briscoe, et al., 2006). Low confidence was expressed from the educators regarding the clinicians' ability to discriminate between weak, failing and excellent medical student performances. Respondents thought that 20–30% of students receiving honours grades reflected grade inflation. Thus, there is a compelling evidence base of belief that some medical students in the US receive grades higher than their practice warrants, especially when the student passed when they should not have.

With regards to the minimum acceptable level in nursing, a theme in the qualitative study was whether the student was 'safe to practice' (Amicucci, 2012). The purposive study of 11 US faculty, explored their lived experience. It was one of only a few qualitative studies that had a theoretical underpinning, thus elevating its credibility. While safety was key, this concept was wide-ranging from 'not killed anyone yet' to 'it is hard to determine who is unsafe' (Amicucci, 2012, p.53). Therefore, there was no cut-off point between acceptable and unacceptable, rather a continuum. The other themes all support the notion of how difficult it is to determine competence and the impact on staff of ending a student's career. The expression giving students the 'benefit of the doubt' encapsulates the wish that students would succeed or 'flunk out', so that faculty did not have to actively fail them (Amicucci, 2012, p.53). This suggests that faculty dislike or avoid using their authority to fail students. The implication of this study is that individual students may benefit from grade inflation, especially those on the border of competence.

Two studies in the review explicitly examined or observed an inflation trend over time (Scanlan and Care, 2004; Roden, 2016). Roden (2016) stated a 1% increase in occupational therapy students' practice grades each year in their five-year study. More recent graduates achieved higher practice grades than their predecessors. Similarly, Scanlan and Care (2004) documented that grade point averages had increased in their Canadian university over the past 25 years, with a statistically significant increase in the grades in the faculty of nursing. Both studies had large samples, they were conducted over time, and their analysis seems robust. Thus, they state limited parity in the practice grades awarded between successive cohorts. However, one could argue that the students were better equipped each year and the increase was not attributed to inflation. Trends towards higher grades over time were also discussed in nursing and midwifery education, although this was not the focus of the research (Hatfield and Lovegrove, 2012; Fisher et al., 2017).

Six studies compared theory and practice grades to show evidence of inflated practice grades (Walsh and Seldomridge, 2005; Susmarini and Hayati, 2011; Edwards, 2012; Hatfield and Lovegrove, 2012; Paskausky and Simonelli, 2014; Roden, 2016). Susmarini and Hayati (2011) interviewed six US nurse educators. As the research set out to explore grade inflation, the implication was that it existed. The researchers did not present evidence to establish how widespread this was; however, they presented practice grades that were close to the maximum point. They expressed a pressure on faculty to award high grades from students and employers alike. As most students passed the course and failed the national licensure examination, they argued that the practice grades were inflated as students did not have the requisite underlying knowledge. They implied that faculty abdicated their responsibility to fail students' practice (Susmarini and Hayati, 2011).

In the UK, Edwards' (2012) evaluation of 38 student midwives grades over one year found that most practice grades were closely clustered. This, she suggested, was due to consistency between mentors. However, she questioned how mentors evaluated the students' practice as some students had significantly lower scores for their underpinning knowledge (Edwards, 2012). Also, in the UK, a nursing study compared previous students' theory and practice grades to establish whether the two were similar (Hatfield and Lovegrove, 2012). The number of student grades was not stated, but 48% of the previous four years' grades were within 10% of each other for theory and practice with the remaining 52% higher for practice. The implication of this is that the relationship between theory and practice grades is limited. While all three of these studies were small, they are supported by larger studies with similar findings (Walsh and Seldomridge, 2005; Roden, 2016).

Walsh and Seldomridge (2005) compared 184 student theory and practice grades in a range of placements; adult, paediatrics, psychiatry and maternity. They noted a normal distribution curve for theory assessments but negative distribution for practice over five years. The mean theory grades ranged from 2.4 to 2.93/4 with mean practice grades higher at 3.3–3.72/4. Their assumption that there should be some relationship between theory and practice grades was not proven. The same finding was also evident in the large study of 1057 occupational therapy student grades where the theory grades were centred around the B/C mark, and the practice grades were on the A/B border (Roden, 2016).

Paskausky and Simonelli (2014) also found a low correlation between theory and practice grades from 281 scores. They too identified a narrow grade distribution for practice but wider for theory assessments and negatively skewed practice grades. They postulated that the evaluation method for practice assessment is likely to cause the reduced range and challenged its validity (Paskausky and Simonelli, 2014). Collectively these six studies reveal a discrepancy between the theory and practice grades across professions, and a limited relationship between underpinning knowledge and practice grades.

One reason for this might be the reluctance by assessors to award grades for knowledge. This was explicitly mentioned in two qualitative studies (Smith, 2007; Hatfield and Lovegrove, 2012). Similarly, midwives were hesitant about assessing students' research understanding, considering this to be the role of the university (Smith, 2007). One could argue that knowledge and evidence-based practice are fundamental to nursing and midwifery practice, even though some assessors did not think that it was part of their role to assess it. An alternative view is that theory and practice are distinct entities and that there is little relationship between the two.

The contribution of the clinical grade to the overall degree classification was discussed in the reviewed literature in three surveys (Briscoe et al., 2006; Fisher et al., 2017; Lawson et al., 2016). In Lawson et al.'s (2016) national study of 100 medical directors, the practice grade contributed to 20–100% of the overall degree. A smaller study in medicine stated that the clinical grade was based on direct observation of practice and this contributed to 50–70% of the final grade (Briscoe et al., 2006). However, the authors do not say how the rest of the grade was derived (Briscoe et al., 2006). In medicine, the final award is a Bachelor of Medicine and/or Surgery, rather than a first, second or third class medical degree, so the impact of grading practice is not as conspicuous as in nursing or midwifery where degree classifications are awarded.

The number of academic credits in midwifery programmes for practice ranged from 10 to 60 out of 120 credits each year; equivalent to 8–50% of the final grade (Fisher et al., 2017). Given that practice grades tend towards the higher ranges, the effect on degree classifications will depend on the weighting between theory and practice assessments within a curriculum. The implication here is that degree classifications between universities even within one profession are not comparable. This demonstrates moderate evidence to suggest marked variation in how much of the practice grade contributes to the overall degree, as the survey consisted of 40 participants with a good response rate (73%) from the total population of 55 Lead Midwives for Education (Fisher et al., 2017).

1.3.2 Student preference: graded or competence assessment

The change from a graded assessment to a binary pass/fail competence assessment was studied by Manning et al. (2016). The change was acceptable to 67 pharmacy students, although the number that were asked is not clear. The students described how they wanted to show ability rather than being motivated by the grade awarded (Manning et al., 2016). The change was not associated with a decrease in motivation or performance of students, which was an early concern from the mentors (n=155 in total). In this study, the students were not given a choice of assessment; they evaluated the change.

When offered the choice of a graded placement or assessment of competence alone, most medical students in one UK study chose the graded placement (Lefroy et al., 2015). Third-year students who agreed to participate were randomised into two groups. The first group received grades on the first placement and a pass/refer mark with feedback on the second and vice versa for group two. Each of these students then chose whether to have a graded final placement. From 144 students, 110 (76%) volunteered; however, only 83 completed the study; 78% of them chose the graded final placement with only 22% preferring no grade. A sample of

24 students were interviewed who explained the reasons for their choices as well as an open-ended question for all students surveyed (Lefroy et al., 2015). There was no clear difference between the groups who chose grading from competence assessment on previous grades, i.e. those who had a borderline pass were not more likely to choose competence assessment. Students said that grades enabled them to locate themselves within their peer group (Lefroy et al., 2015). However, some students thought that qualitative feedback was more powerful than the grade itself (Lefroy et al., 2015). One could argue that the grade is a symbol that does not in itself offer any information, especially if almost all students receive high grades, rather it is the interpretation students and assessors alike place on the grade. Students said the grades could increase their effort or affect their self-confidence and/or self-efficacy and were sometimes attributed to the relationship between the mentor and student (Lefroy et al., 2015).

Not all students agreed with their grades and this had a negative effect on them (Lefroy et al., 2015). Therefore, the process of grading practice was not positive for all students and depended on a positive mentoring relationship. Consideration of the mentoring relationship, its effect on student learning and the grading process was largely missing from the quantitative studies. However, it was a major feature in the qualitative studies and will be considered in more depth later. It seems that learning in clinical practice and its assessments is essentially a social interaction between students and assessors.

1.4 Issues with grading practice

The two most frequently cited issues with grading students' practice are feedback and lack of time. Compliance with feedback in medical education has already been identified as an issue and discussed (Hiller et al., 2016; Lawson et al., 2016). Similarly, the quality of feedback in nursing, especially good quality constructive negative feedback enabled students to evaluate their practice more accurately than positive feedback (Plakht et al., 2013).

Heaslip and Scammell (2012), in the introduction to phase three of their three-year service evaluation, argued that binary competence assessments (pass/fail) provided limited feedback to students on their performance, thus implying that grading practice is superior. Their convenience sample of 107 students and 112 mentors were accessed through tutor groups and a mentor conference, respectively. The higher response rate (86%) for mentors may indicate that there was an expectation to participate in the research at the conference. Only 51% of the final-year students participated. However, as this was the third of three phases, there may have been an element of research fatigue if the same students were sampled previously, which may have happened (Scammell et al., 2007).

The students and mentors in the Heaslip and Scammell (2012) study had divergent views on feedback from practice; 92% of mentors thought that they delivered this effectively throughout the placement. However, 56% of students said that they only received feedback at the end of the placement. Three formal meetings were scheduled during each placement between the student and mentor, yet 12.5% of students said that they did not receive any feedback at all (Heaslip and Scammell, 2012). When asked whether the feedback matched the grade awarded, 89% of mentors agreed that it did, while only 60% of students felt this way. A discrepancy between qualitative feedback and practice grades were also noted in the national midwifery study (Fisher et al., 2017). The implication here could be that mentors have difficulty offering face-to-face feedback to students, especially if the feedback needed is constructive criticism. Simultaneously, perhaps students do not recognise they are receiving feedback.

Two national surveys in medicine cite reluctance to give negative or candid feedback to students (Briscoe et al., 2006; Fazio et al., 2013). Both studies had reasonable sample sizes, and their recruitment strategy suggested that they were likely to be representative, thus increasing the weight of evidence. Medical directors in Fazio et al.'s (2013) survey admitted that they avoided dealing with unhappy, upset or angry students in 27% of responses; it was the most common response and a potential source of grade inflation. Their discussion postulated that face-to-face feedback, especially avoiding giving negative feedback, contributed to grade inflation. Briscoe et al.'s (2006) survey demonstrated low confidence levels in doctors' ability to discriminate between student performances and ascribed some of this to the difficulty of giving candid feedback to students. One can postulate that the lack of negative feedback means that assessors feel a pressure to give high practice grades, as noted earlier, for fear of potential conflict from the students. This reinforces the notion that the practice grades are imprecise, or at least imprecise for some students and that some students may be able to influence the grade awarded.

1.4.1 Lack of time for grading practice

Time was measured in two studies grading physiotherapy students' practice (Dalton et al., 2009; Murphy et al., 2014). The findings of Dalton et al.'s (2009) large-scale action research project undertaken over multiple university sites with numerous stakeholders to test a new assessment tool is supported by Murphy et al.'s (2014) smaller study. On average, Dalton et al.'s (2009) grading tool took 17–28 minutes for mentors to administer. This was acceptable to the assessors and students alike. Murphy et al.'s (2014) study, which compared the change from one grading tool to another took 23 minutes (with a standard deviation of 13) to complete. This was reduced from the older tool which required 80 minutes (and a wide standard deviation of 53 minutes). Most of the 80 students (82%) preferred the newer faster assessment, despite a slight reduction in practice grades (from 84% to 78%) (Murphy et al., 2014). While both tools were positively evaluated, the authors made no reference to the pressures of time in clinical practice to explain how this may have affected the participants' views.

The qualitative studies tended to discuss the lack of time for education in clinical practice in the UK and USA which impacted university staff and clinicians' ability to grade practice (Hanley and Higgins, 2005; Walsh and Seldomridge, 2005; Smith, 2007; Susmarini and Hayati, 2011). Susmarini and Hayati's (2011) study of six faculty who were expected to work with students three times per week admitted spending only 15–20 minutes of time once per week with individual students. Anecdotal records reported in Walsh and Seldomridge's (2005) study said that faculty were unable to maintain accurate student records due to time constraints. Mentors in Smith's (2007) small scale study said that they were unable to devote as much time as they would like to supporting students due to the pressure of work. This is further corroborated by students in Hanley and Higgins (2005) qualitative study who suggested that assessors needed more time to observe the students' practice. Collectively these studies suggest that the time for observation, teaching and assessment in clinical practice is limited, which is likely to influence the quality of feedback and accuracy of the grade awarded.

1.5 Problematising the research: practice assessment as social interactions

Dictionary definitions of assessment tend to focus on value or quality; the act of assessing, appraising or evaluating (Walsh, 2010). However, there are many variables depending on who and what is being assessed; which have been considered above. Rowntree (1987, p. 4) sees assessment 'occurring when one person, in some kind of interaction, direct or indirect, with another, is conscious of obtaining and interpreting information about the knowledge and understanding, or abilities and attitudes of that other person'. In his words, it is to 'know' that person.

Examining the effect of the relationship between the student and mentor in practice is essential to understanding the assessment. While each pedagogic relationship is unique, they will share common characteristics. The assessment outcome says something about the students' work but also about their relationships with others (Schostak et al., 1994). The student who knows not to 'rock the boat' is likely to make the 'right' impression with their mentor (Clouder, 2003). These students, who understand their interactions, are more likely to be successful. The problem then with pedagogic relationships and assessment is to enable all students to understand their interactions and the significance of these on the relationship with others and the assessment practices.

Many studies noted the special and supportive relationship between students and assessors in clinical practice. Some mentors were aware of the relationship that they developed with the student, recognising if the student mirrored their way of working this positively affected the grade. Similarly, the relationship hindered delivering candid feedback and leniency in grading seemed to occur (Briscoe et al., 2006; Seldomridge and Walsh, 2006; Fazio et al., 2013). Assigning lower grades was more difficult when the boundary between student and faculty was blurred and an emotional bond had developed (Scanlan and Care, 2004). One study suggested investigating the relationship between the student and placement educator, which was hypothesised to impact upon the assessment of practice (Roden, 2016).

One way to increase the reliability and validity of the practice assessment was to 'separate out the relationship' that developed over several weeks in clinical practice (Clouder and Toms, 2008). One student in this study perceived that the grade awarded for practice was dependent upon the quality of interactions with the practice educator and that the oral exam assessed by two people was more objective than the mentor only assessment (Clouder and Toms, 2008). A lack of relationship with an assessor was interpreted to have an impact on a student's confidence, and this was attributed to a low practice grade (Lefroy et al., 2015).

To bring together the distinct types of practice assessments, Wolff (2007) offers a discourse on grading. He refers to grading compulsory education in the USA, but many of the principles apply equally to healthcare education programmes. In his 'ideal university', Wolff defines three types of grading: criticism, evaluation and ranking. Criticism, when used to assess complex matters, such as healthcare, is bound up in arguments over style. A mentor who has one style may prefer the student to adopt a similar style; commensurate with the mentor's normative values. Smith's (2007) midwifery study acknowledged this halo effect. Some sort of evaluative standard may be implicit in the criticism grade, but not always. If a student's style is not commensurate with the mentors' values and beliefs, there will be tension within this form of grading.

Evaluation, the second type of grading, is the measuring of a performance against a standard of excellence (Wolff, 2007). There is an association between competence and standards (Norris, 1991). The standard is a desirable or necessary level of attainment. It should be possible to determine whether a student's practice is acceptable or unacceptable. However, some of the studies were not able to discriminate between pass and fail performances (Reubenson et al., 2012; Eggleton et al., 2016). According to Wolff, it is possible to determine excellent, acceptable or unacceptable performances but not to provide a linear scale of grades from 0 to 100 as this is too fine a measurement for accurate discrimination. While several studies had three or four descriptors (Seldomridge and Walsh, 2006; Pulito et al., 2007; Murphy et al., 2014; Lefroy et al., 2015) many of the practice grades stated were expressed as a percentage (for example, Plakht et al., 2013; Murphy et al., 2014; Hiller et al., 2016). Therefore, one can question the accuracy of these grades, especially when most grades were in the 70%+ bracket (Table 1.2). The grades seem to signify something but not necessarily a measure of performance against the criteria because according to Wolff (2007) it is not possible to be that accurate.

Ranking is the third grading activity, where a mentor considers the performance of this student on the merits of the predecessor, which is whether this student is better or worse than the last student (Wolff, 2007). This form of grading does not allow the mentor to demonstrate how much better this student is and should not be used in healthcare education, since each student should be assessed on their merits against an acceptable standard that protects the public. Wolff supports this premise, stating that evaluation is at the heart of professional practice (Wolff, 2007). A pass means that the healthcare student can enter the professional register; a fail means they cannot. Wolff suggests that since most professions are now degree educated, educators should dispense with the grading of practice and award the degree and eligibility to enter the profession upon meeting the standards alone. However, this is clearly not what is happening from the research (Table 1.2).

1.5.1 Why does this matter?

Figure 1.1 illustrates the findings from the literature review. This sits inside Figure 1.2, which has the scope to consider the wider challenges the midwifery profession in the UK currently faces. Challenges need to be acknowledged as they have an effect on the education of midwifery students, the midwives working in a stretched environment and the women who access the maternity services. The Royal College of Midwives, the professional body and trade union for most midwives in the UK, reports on the State of Maternity Services (RCM, 2015; RCM, 2018). While the numbers of midwives working in England has

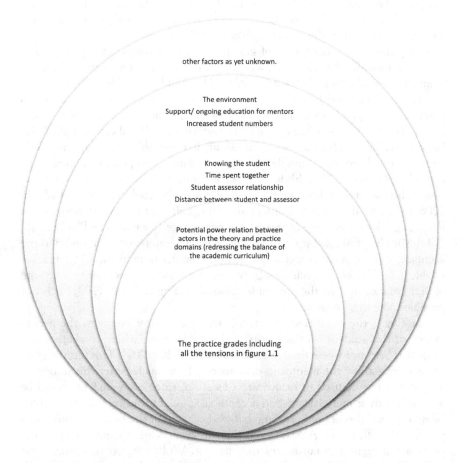

other factors as yet unknown.

The environment
Support/ ongoing education for mentors
Increased student numbers

Knowing the student
Time spent together
Student assessor relationship
Distance between student and assessor

Potential power relation between
actors in the theory and practice
domains (redressing the balance of
the academic curriculum)

The practice grades including
all the tensions in figure 1.1

Figure 1.2 Visual representation of the qualitative findings; the wider context of grading clinical practice.

risen since 2010, the number of midwives over 50 years old is still a concern as this population is close to retirement. This means that more students need to be educated to replace these midwives so the newly qualified staff have time to develop experience.

While the number of births in England and Wales in 2019 has reduced to 640,370 (ONS, 2020) from its high of almost 700,000 in 2012, the age profile of women using maternity services continues to increase (RCM, 2018), with 55% of births to women in their thirties or higher in England. Women who give birth later in life may need more care which adds to the pressure on the service. This coupled with the rising level of obesity means that more midwives are needed to deliver the service (RCM, 2018). England has been commissioning approximately 2500 student midwives per year; however, only 2000 of these graduate annually, which is a 51% increase from 2010/2011. While this number would appear to improve the country's shortfall of 3500 midwives, the NMC register saw a net increase of only 67 full-time midwives in 2018 (ibid.). The number of EU trained midwives coming to work in the UK also reduced dramatically following the UK referendum (RCM, 2018). Moreover, in 2017 changes to the funding stream for student midwives meant that the number of applicants to the profession dropped. Future student numbers are unknown despite the re-introduction of a bursary for September 2020 onwards. While these concerns affect the current workforce, they have been affecting the workforce and provision of care for the last decade. It is during this timeframe that this research was conducted, focusing on the introduction of grading of practice to midwifery education from 2009, with these challenges in the background.

1.6 A gap in the literature and research questions

From the literature, a gap is noted in the potential effect of the relationship between students and midwives and how this may affect the practice grade. Issues that seemed to compromise the reliability of the practice grade were compliance with formative or summative feedback to students, assessors' ability or authority to give candid feedback or grades to students, differences in understanding what the grade signified and whether observation of a student's practice alone was a reliable method on which to base a grade. Additionally, the reviewed literature lacked a theoretical or conceptual base. Thus, my research will aim to fill these gaps. The research questions stemmed from the critiqued literature, endeavour to explore:

1. What counts as valid midwifery practice knowledge?
2. What meaning do students and mentors attribute to the practice grade?
3. Is there a difference, real or perceived, between the quantitative grades awarded and qualitative feedback given to students?
4. What else is happening in the interactions between students and mentors that may be affecting the relationship or grade?

To fulfil the traditions of a qualitative study, the assessment of practice will not be isolated from the process of students learning and the nature of the assessment. The organic nature of qualitative research meant that I needed to respond to the complexities of the site and the participants. Therefore, I drew on further literature on what counts as valid knowledge in midwifery practice and teaching, learning and mentorship in clinical practice to support the interpretation of findings and discussions. To research the topic, I chose to include multiple methods of data collection in a case study approach. I listened to various stakeholders, which included students, mentors and other lecturers' viewpoints and reviewed the students' grades and practice assessment documents.

The methodology and philosophical underpinnings of the project are explained in the next chapter. The phenomenon of grading students' midwifery practice was informed by the work of Basil Bernstein and his theorisation of power and control in the transmission and validation of educational knowledge. The research is qualitative in nature and considers assessment as a social, relational phenomenon. This perspective has also been used to reflect upon my dual roles as researcher and lecturer.

Bibliography

Amicucci, B., (2012). What nurse faculty have to say about clinical grading. *Teaching and Learning in Nursing*, 7(2), pp. 51–55.

Bhugra, D. & Malik, A., (2011). *Workplace-Based Assessments in Psychiatric Training*. Cambridge: Cambridge University Press.

Briscoe, G. W. Carlson, D. L, Arcand, L. A, Levine, R. E. & Cohen, M. J., (2006). Clinical grading in psychiatric clerkships. *Academic Psychiatry*, 30(2), pp. 104–109.

Bryar, R. & Sinclair, M., (2011). *Theory for Midwifery Practice*. 2nd ed. Basingstoke: Palgrave Macmillan Ltd.

Clouder, L., (2003). Becoming professional; exploring the complexities of professional socialisation in health and social care. *Learning in Health and Social Care*, 2(4), pp. 213–222.

Clouder, L. & Toms, J., (2008). Impact of oral assessment on physiotherapy 'students' learning in practice. *Physiotherapy Theory and Practice*, 24(1), pp. 29–42.

Dalton, M., Keating, J. & Davidson, M., (2009). *Development of the Assessment of Physiotherapy Practice (APP): A Standardised and Valid Approach to Assessment of Clinical Competence in Physiotherapy*. s.l.: Australian Learning and Teaching Council (ALTC) Final report.

Docherty, A. & Dieckmann, N., (2015). Is there evidence of failing to fail in our schools of nursing? *Nursing Education Perspectives*, 36(4), pp. 226–231.

Donaldson, J. & Gray, M., (2012). Systematic review of grading practice: Is there evidence of grade inflation? *Nurse Education in Practice*, 12(2), pp. 101–114.

Duffy, K., (2004). *A Grounded Theory Investigation of Factors Which Influence the Assessment of Students' Competence to Practice*. London: Nursing and Midwifery Council.

Edwards, A., (2012). Grading practice: An evaluation one year on. *Nurse Education Today*, 32(6), pp. 627–629.

Eggleton, K., Goodyear-Smith, F., Paton, L., Fallon, K., Wong, C., Lack, L., Kennelly, J., Fishman, T. & Moyes, S., (2016). Reliability of mini-CEX assessment of medical students in general practice clinical attachments. *Family Medicines*, 48(8), p. 624.

Eraut, M., (1994). *Developing Professional Knowledge and Competence*. Abingdon: Routledge.

Fazio, S. B., Papp, K. K., Torre, D. M. & DeFer, T. M., (2013). Grade inflation in the internal medicine clerkship: A national survey. *Teaching and Learning in Medicine*, 25(1), pp. 71–76.

Fisher, M., Bower, H., Chenery-Morris, S., Jackson, J. & Way, S., (2017). A scoping study to explore the application and impact of grading practice in pre-registration midwifery programmes across the United Kingdom. *Nurse Education in Practice*, 24, pp. 99–105.

Fraser, D., Avis, M. & Mallik, M., (2013). The MINT project- An evaluation of the impact of midwife teachers on the outcomes of pre-registration midwifery education in the UK. *Midwifery*, 29, pp. 86–94.

Fraser, D. M., (1988). *Preparing Effective Midwives: An Outcome Evaluation of the Effectiveness of Pre-Registration Midwifery Programmes of Education*. London: English National Board.

Girot, E., (1993). Assessment of competence in clinical practice-a review of the literature. *Nurse Education Today*, 13(2), pp. 83–90.

Gray, M. & Donaldson, J., (2009a). *Exploring Issues in the Use of Grading in Practice; Literature Review Final Report Volume 1*. Edinburgh: Edinburgh Napier University.

Gray, M. & Donaldson, J., (2009b). *Exploring Issues in the Use of Grading in Practice; Literature Review Final Report Volume 2*. Edinburgh: Edinburgh Napier University.

Hanley, E. & Higgins, A., (2005). Assessment of practice in intensive care: Students' perceptions of a clinical competence assessment tool. *Intensive and Critical Care Nursing*, 21(5), pp. 276–283.

Hart, C., (1988). *Doing a Literature Review Releasing the Social Science Research Imagination*. London: SAGE Ltd.

Hatfield, D. & Lovegrove, J., (2012). The use of skills inventories to assess and grade practice: Part 2. *Evaluation of Assessment Strategy*, 12(3), pp. 133–138.

Heaslip, V. & Scammell, J. M., (2012). Failing underperforming students: The role of grading in practice assessment. *Nurse Education in Practice*, 12(2), pp. 95–100.

Hiller, K. M., Waterbrook, A. & Waters, K., (2016). Timing of emergency medicine student evaluation does not affect scoring. *Journal of Emergency Medicine*, 50(2), pp. 302–307.

Hunt, L. A., McGee, P., Gutteridge, R. & Hughes, M., (2016). Failing securely; the processes and support which underpin English nurse mentors' assessment decisions regarding under-performing students. *Nurse Education Today*, 39, pp. 79–86.

ICM, (2017). *Midwifery: An Autonomous Profession*. Toronto: International Confederation of Midwives.

Imanipour, M. & Jalili, M., (2016). Development of a comprehensive clinical performance assessment system for nursing students: A programmatic approach. *Japan Journal of Nursing Science*, 13(1), pp. 46–54.

Larocque, S. & Luhanga, F., (2013). Exploring the issue of failure to fail in a nursing program. *International Journal of Nursing Education Scholarship*, 10(1), pp. 1–8.

Lawson, L., Jung, J. & Hiller, K., (2016). Clinical assessment of medical students in emergency medicine clerkships: A survey of current practice. *Journal of Emergency Medicine*, 51(6), pp. 705–711.

Lefroy, J., Hawarden, A., Gay, S., McKinley, R. K & Cleland, J., (2015). Grades in formative workplace-based assessment: A study of what works for whom and why. *Medical Education*, 49(3), pp. 307–320.

Luhanga, F., Yonge, O. & Myrick, F.,(2008). Failure to assign failing grades: Issues with grading the unsafe student. *International Journal of Nursing Education Scholarship*, 5(1), pp. 1–13.

Lurie, S. J. & Mooney, C. J., (2010). Relationship between clinical assessment and examination scores in determining clerkship grade. *Medical Education*, 44(2), pp. 177–183.

Manning, D. H., Ference, K. A., Welch, A. C. & Holt-Macey, M., (2016). Development and implementation of pass/fail grading system for advanced pharmacy practice experiences. *Americal Journal of Pharmaceutical Education*, 8(1), pp. 59–68.

McGregor, A., (2007). Academic success, clinical failure: Struggling practices of a failing student. *Journal of Nursing Education*, 46(11), pp. 504–511.

Meldrum, D., Lydon, A. M., Loughnane, M., Geary, F., Shanley, L., Sayers, K., Shinnick, E. & Filan, D., (2008). Assessment of undergraduate physiotherapist clinical performance: Investigation of educator inter-rater reliability. *Physiotherapy*, 94(3), pp. 212–219.

Miller, G., (1990). The assessment of clinical skills/ competence/ performance. *Academic Medicine*, 65(9), pp. s63–67.

Murphy, S., Dalton, M. & Dawes, D., (2014). Assessing physical therapy students' performance during clinical practice. *Physiotherapy Canada*, 66(2), pp. 169–176.

NMC, (2006). NMC Consultation, '*Review of Pre-Registration Midwifery Education*', *Decisions*. London: Nursing and Midwifery Council.

NMC, (2008). *Standards to Support Learning and Assessment in Practice*. London: Nursing and Midwifery Council.

NMC, (2009). *Standards for Pre-Registration Midwifery Education*. London: Nursing and Midwifery Council.

NMC, (2010). *Standards of Pre-Registration Nursing Education*. London: Nursing and Midwifery Council.

NMC, (2018a). *Standards for Pre-Registration Nursing Programmes*. London: Nursing and Midwifery Council.

NMC, (2018b). *The Code Professional Standards of Practice and Behaviour for Nurses, Midwives and Nursing Associates*. London: Nursing and Midwifery Council.

NMC, (2019). *Standards for Pre-Registration Midwifery Programmes*. London: Nursing and Midwifery Council.

Norris, N., (1991). The trouble with competence. *Cambridge Journal of Education*, 21(3), pp. 331–341.

Oermann, M., Yarborough, S. S., Saewert, K. J., Ard, N. & Charasika, M., (2009). Clinical evaluation and grading practices in schools of nursing; national survey findings part 2. *Nursing Education Perspectives*, 30(6), pp. 352–357.

ONS, (2020). *Births in England and Wales: 2019*. London: Office for National Statistics.

Paskausky, A. L. & Simonelli, M. C., (2014). Measuring grade inflation: A clinical grade discrepancy score. *Nurse Education in Practice*, 14(4), pp. 374–379.

Plakht, Y., Shiyovich, A., Nusbaum, L. & Raizer, H., (2013). The association of positive and negative feedback with clinical performance, self-evaluation and practice contribution of nursing students. *Nurse Education Today*, 33(10), pp. 1264–1268.

Pulito, A. R., Donnelly, M. B. & Plymale, M., (2007). Factors in faculty evaluation of medical students' performance. *Medical Education*, 41(7), pp. 667–675.

RCM, (2015). *State of Maternity Services Report 2015*. London: Royal College of Midwives.

RCM, (2018). *State of Maternity Services Report 2018*. London: Royal College of Midwives.

Reubenson, A., Schnepf, T., Waller, R. & Edmondson, S., (2012). Inter-examiner agreement in clinical evaluation. *The Clinical Teacher*, 9(2), pp. 119–122.

Ridely, D., (2008). *A Literature Review A Step by Step Guide for Students*. London: SAGE Ltd.

Roden, P., (2016). Do occupational therapy graduates benefit from grade inflation on practice placements? *British Journal of Occupational Therapy*, 77(3), pp. 134–138.

Rowntree, D., (1987). *Assessing Students; How Shall We Know Them*. London: Kogan Page Ltd.

Scammell, J., Halliwell, D. & Partlow, C., (2007). *Assessment of Practice in Pre-Registration Undergraduate Nursing Programmes: An Evaluation of a Tool to Grade Student Performance in Practice*. Bournemouth: Bournemouth University.

Scanlan, J. M. & Care, W. D., (2004). Grade inflation: Should we be concerned? *Journal of Nursing Education*, 43(10), pp. 475–478.

Scanlan, J. M. & Chernomas, W. M., (2016). Failing clinical practice and the unsafe student: A new perspective. *International Journal of Education Scholarship*, 13(1), pp. 109–116.

Schostak, J. et al., (1994). *The ACE Project: The Assessment of Competence in Nursing and Midwifery*, London: English National Board for Nursing, Midwifery and Health Visiting.

Seldomridge, L. A. & Walsh, C. M., (2006). Evaluating student performance in undergraduate preceptorships. *Journal of Nursing Education*, 45(5), pp. 169–176.

Smith, J., (2007). Assessing and grading students' clinical practice: Midwives lived experience. *Evidence Based Midwifery*, 5(4), pp. 112–119.

Susmarini, D. & Hayati, Y. S., (2011). Grade inflation in clinical stage. *American Journal of Health Sciences*, 2(1), p. 21.

Walsh, C. M. & Seldomridge, L. A., (2005). Clinical grades: Upward bound. *Journal of Nursing Education*, 44(4), pp. 162–168.

Walsh, D., (2010). *The Nurse 'Mentor's Handbook Supporting Students in Clinical Practice*. Maidenhead: Open University Press.

Weaver, C. S., Humbert, A. J., Besinger, B. R., Graber, J. A. & Brizendine, E. J., (2007). A more explicit grading scale decreases grade inflation in a clinical clerkship. *Academic Emergency Medicine*, 14(3), pp. 283–286.

Wolff, R. P., (2007). A discourse on grading. In: R. Curren, ed. *Philosophy of Education*. Oxford: Blackwell Publishing Ltd, pp. 489–464.

2 Methodology

The assessment of students' practice is not a clearly defined, measurable, objective fact and, as such, there are multiple perspectives to consider rather than one single reality. Therefore, the interpretive approach offered a great deal for studying this phenomenon (Denzin, 2001). As an interpretive researcher, I assumed that access to these realities was enabled through social constructions such as language and shared meaning (Denzin, 2001). I needed to appreciate the differences between people in focussing on different meanings. The aim of this research was to explore the effects of grading practices on students, mentors, and lecturers' relationships, identities, and authorities. Therefore, I had to explore the experiences and ideas expressed in participants' narrative accounts, and take a stance in relation to the meaning of their practices. I needed to know about and know how grading affected the individuals, and potentially, the profession.

The two distinct forms of epistemological knowledge are 'knowing about' and 'knowing how'. Eraut (1994) called them propositional and practical knowledge, respectively. Propositional knowledge underpins or enables professionals to act, while practical knowledge is the action itself and cannot be separated from propositional knowledge (Eraut, 1994, p.15). However, in Carper's (1978) seminal text on patterns of knowing in nursing, four types of knowledge were named: empirics, the science of nursing; (a)esthetics, the art of nursing; ethics, the moral component; and personal knowledge. Empirics is 'knowing about' nursing, whereas aesthetic knowledge is particular rather than general knowledge which is the 'how to' element. This is, according to Carper, more difficult to explain than scientific knowledge. Eraut (1994) supports this saying that tacit or practical knowledge is difficult to articulate. The art of nursing is observed in action, in the style of care delivered in the empathy and perception of the patient's needs. This is intricately linked to personal knowledge, not only of the self but of the other, but in the interactions, relationships, and transactions between nurses and their patients; in therapeutic relationships (Carper, 1978). Each of the four elements is separate but interrelated and interdependent.

In terms of this study, therefore, it would be difficult to separate 'knowing about' midwifery practice from 'knowing how' to practise midwifery. Similarly, knowing about midwifery practice cannot really be separated from how this knowledge is acquired. By this I mean how I researched the topic; the actions and decisions I took are an integral part of the knowledge generated, and the findings cannot be disconnected from the act of the research or researcher. Knowledge generated this way raises questions about the nature of objectivity in research and between subject and object.

Objectivity in research is seen as crucial to the quality of research which assumes truth can be determined as something distinct from a particular person or context. It refers to the removal of the person, their emotions, knowledge, and values, from the research process (Somekh and Lewin, 2011, p.326). When the aim of a study is to explore how drugs interact with the body or whether one method of suturing is superior to another, it is possible to research these areas objectively, without a problem. However, when research focuses on a social phenomenon, such as grading practices, this is not the case.

In the study of knowledge, subject and object are crucial epistemological components. Subject refers to an active, conscious individual or social group with an intent, while object refers to the way the subject thinks or acts (Christiensen and James, 2008). The object of my study can be perceived in several ways. It is the grades, the grading practices, and the meanings derived from these by the subjects. The object is not a passive, discrete object; it is socially constructed. The meanings cannot be understood in isolation from the subjects' experiences. Therefore, grading practices can be understood as socially produced objects. The meanings derived by each group of participants, as this is preferred to the word subject, as it conveys less dominance by the researcher, are likely to differ according to the participant's positioning (Somekh and Lewin, 2011). Therefore, the inclusion of different participants was necessary to represent the various perspectives offered by participants of the same object, and a qualitative approach was needed.

Due to the interactive nature of learning in clinical practice, one conceptual framework considered for this study was interactionism (Denzin, 2001). Interactionism can be understood as the narrow branch of symbolic interactionism but equally as a more broad study of social encounters such as face-to-face interaction, the construction of self and identity, and knowledge in social groups and institutions (Atkinson and Housley, 2003). Interactionism offers qualitative researchers the ability to capture the unique experiences of diverse members of a community. In this project, the experiences of students, mentors, and lecturers interacting to producing the next generation of midwives through knowledge transmission, professional socialisation, and assessments were considered.

The interactions in midwifery education and practice, the object of this study, are, however, part of an overall system or structure of relations that occur in large social organisations. The structural or hierarchical nature of midwifery education in the UK and abroad and low status of students and junior staff have been identified by others (Deery, 2005; Begley, 2001, 2002; Fenwick et al., 2012; Hunter, 2005). The cited research explored student, newly qualified, and experienced midwives' experiences of working in maternity systems in the UK, Ireland, and Australia. The structure, especially within the hospital environment, affected the integration of individuals into the profession. For some, the structure was evident; for instance, students 'knew their place' (Begley, 2001). For others, including newly qualified midwives, this was less evident, facilitated by positive midwife-to-midwife interactions to enable a more supportive integration into midwifery. However, conflict has been described between junior and senior midwives and between hospital and community staff (Hunter, 2005). Thus, the structural relations cannot be ignored as they affect the student, mentor, and lecturers differently.

Individuals' status and relationships with others will affect what the participants say and mean, not only in the collection of their experiences but also in their interactions within clinical practice. It is this rich mix of macro and microsocial practices that I aimed to understand to explore grading practices. The interactionist perspective was suitable as a conceptual framework for the microsocial features of the study. However, interactionism is not able to encompass the status and structure of the workplace for the participants. Therefore, a general interactionist stance was used as well as a specific theory.

During the research, several theoretical perspectives were considered; these included Gee (2000) and van Vuuren and Westerhof's (2015) analytical frameworks of identity in educational and professional lives. However, after tentative attempts to apply the theory to the empirical data it was clear to me that these were not the right theories for my study because they did not enable a consideration of the structural relations between students and midwives. Similarly, I considered using Benner's (2001) novice to expert framework and Carper's (1978) fundamental patterns in nursing, but neither theory offered a language for the structural relations in practice.

The specific theoretical application comes from Bernstein's (2000) pedagogic codes. The concepts of classification and framing refer to the structural relations and interactional practices, respectively. The concepts create links between the macro structures and micro interactional communicative practices (Bernstein, 2000).

2.1 Bernstein's theories

Basil Bernstein's theories of formal educational knowledge, developed over four decades, are structuralist but draw on Durkheim and interactionism. Bernstein understood Durkheim through the British school of social anthropology; therefore, his reading of Durkheim was informed from this perspective instead of through the more common sociology of education reading (Moore, 2013). Bernstein understood Durkheim's theory of pedagogy from a position at the opposite end of the spectrum from the sociology of education. Hence, to understand Bernstein, one must appreciate his reading of Durkheim. Both Durkheim and Bernstein come to 'the field' with questions that reflect 'deep problems' (Collins, 2000). They believed, the problem is the starting tenet around which resources, theories, and methodologies, are mobilised. The problem comes before the approach (Moore, 2013). According to Moore (2013, p.33):

> Bernstein took from Durkheim the fundamental question; how do human beings become social beings? What is the relationship between the symbolic orders, social relations and experience, between the inner and outer?

Expressed most simply, the origins of inner and outer come from Kant (Pickering, 2000). Reality is made up of experiences inside and outside the individual (Pickering, 2000). This is analogous to Carper's (1978) types of knowledge and knowing the self to know another. Durkheim's take on the concepts was related to religion (Sandovnik, 1995). Sacred religious knowledge, the outer, was set apart from society and removed from everyday life, the inner, or profane. The distinction between the inner and outer had its roots in the social division of labour. However, Durkheim explained science which was not sacred could become so by forsaking other knowledge. Bernstein differed in his reading and understands inner and outer as able to co-exist within individuals. The inner person is sacred, and the outer social world is profane. There is always a range of possibilities.

Moore (in the foreword of Frandji and Vitale, 2011) considers Bernstein presented a problematic rather than a theory. Similarly, Bernstein rejected the term paradigm, and preferred the term problematic (Moore, 2013). Bernstein disliked paradigms because they have an incommensurable number of theories, methodologies, and perspectives that cannot 'speak' to each other because they come from different standpoints and are therefore incompatible. He also believed the problematic is a problem field in which many people work together. He rejected the idea that any theory could be a total theory because the social world is always changing, and there can never be theoretical closure. This is significant as Bernstein wanted to identify unfamiliar problems and open them for discussion rather than closing them to focus on the solution. The 'deep problem is the very nature of the social' (Moore, 2013, p.4), in this way interactionism is a relevant theory in that it attempts to make the meanings that circulate in the world of lived experience accessible to the reader (Denzin, 2001, p.1).

According to Atkinson (1985, p.1), Bernstein was one of the 'most influential of British sociologists'. However, his theories of language codes and pedagogic discourses and practices have been misunderstood either by an over-simplistic or partial interpretation of his work, and this has led to criticisms (Moore, 2013). The case of language codes, elaborated and restricted, caused controversy as they were interpreted to be about middle- and working-class communication, respectively, instead of different modalities of communication in differing contexts (Atkinson, 1985; Danzig, 1995; Rosen, 1972). Similarly, Harker and May (1993) considered that Bourdieu provided a more flexible approach than Bernstein to the structure/agency problem. However, Bernstein (2000) responded to this criticism as misrecognition of his work. A further criticism by King (1976) stated that Bernstein's work lacked empirical testing. However, his work was rooted in empirical data and has since been tested by many others (Atkinson, 1985; Moore, 2013), including in vocational and higher education (Muller et al., 2004).

Bernstein's work combined empirical and theoretical work on language and the relationship between language and educational achievement; he strove to analyse disadvantage in the educational system. His work progressed over time and has theorised about the curriculum and school organisation. Due to his extensive career and the development of ever more intricate and re-explained theories, even admirers of his work such as Atkinson (1985), Moore (2013), and Muller

(2006) say his work is incomplete. The restricted and elaborated language codes, for instance, were developed into the terms classification and framing, which will be further explained. Muller considered Bernstein's theory of knowledge structures, particularly those with a weak grammar, such as nursing, is unfinished (Muller, 2006). However, Moore (2013) suggests that this returning to theories and development over time is one of the strengths of his work.

Bernstein's experience as a Jew in London after the Second World War led to his interest in 'structure and the process of cultural transformation' (Atkinson, 1985 p.11). His experience of being an insider and an outsider, member and stranger, led to his appreciation of symbolic boundaries. The role of the personal experience of values, controls and rituals, and the symbolic order in everyday life, and how these are interpreted by individuals, especially when they move into a new educational environment, lies behind his theories or problematics.

Bernstein wanted to:

> develop a sociological framework within which to understand speech as a social as well as a linguistic phenomenon. The problem was how to systematically conceptualise social structure as a mediator between language and speech.
>
> (Moore, 2013, p.58)

Two main theories used within this book are the pedagogic discourse and the pedagogic device. Bernstein understood discourse as a modality of education. Discourses are produced, reproduced, exchanged, distinguished, and appropriated by education (Bernstein, 1990). The social division of labour categorises social relations within the production and between the categories. Within midwifery education, the social division of labour categorises midwives as transmitters and students as acquirers of midwifery knowledge and discourse. The social relations refer to the practices between the transmitters and acquirers – between the midwives and students.

Pedagogic discourses refer to the educational transmission code, how students gain access to knowledge. Differing social groups are orientated to universalistic or particularistic meanings; the linguistic realisation of these two meanings are different. There are two discourses which orientate the learner to meaning. In educational processes, teachers expand the meanings to orientate learners to understand; once a meaning is understood, a less expanded speech pattern can be used. The process of explaining occurs in relationships between acquirers and transmitters. All member of all social groups employ particularistic and universalistic principles according to the context they are in. Between this language and speech there is a social structure. Social structure translates into context, and context in turn can be understood by the terms classification and framing (Moore, 2013, p.63).

The pedagogic discourse introduces the terms classification and framing (Bernstein, 1977). Classification refers to the relationship between categories, whether the categories are between agencies, between agents, between discourses, or between practices. If the categories are well insulated from each other, or clearly separate, the term Bernstein uses is *strong classification* (Bernstein, 1990). When the boundary between categories is blurred, the term is *weak classification* (ibid). Framing refers to the specific pedagogic relationship between the student and teacher; it can also be used between the midwife and woman. Framing is the means of acquiring a legitimate message; this too can be strong or weak. When the teacher is in explicit control over the selection, pacing, and timing of knowledge transmission, the framing is strong. When there is a choice for the student over these aspects of their learning, the framing is weak (Bernstein, 1977). Framing is about who controls what.

Pedagogic discourses are like mazes (Moore, 2013). Different social groups enter mazes through different entrances, but all need to get to the goal, or symbolic meaning. Some may move swiftly to the goal; others take longer, and some may not accomplish the goal. Teachers are the guides through the mazes, but often it is not clear which path is necessary for each student. This is essentially the problematic of the pedagogical discourse. Formal educational contexts are specialised by an elaborating orientation; acquirers need to be able to recognise the specialised context so they can realise an appropriate text within that context. The capability to recognise and realise the specialised context is socially distributed and this means that not all students have equal access to the orientation of meanings; however, teachers can vary their teaching, so all learners acquire the requisite knowledge.

The pedagogic discourse is related to the pedagogic device. The pedagogic device controls who gets what and how: the form and distribution of knowledge (Bernstein, 2000). The device is 'like a field of forces' it is a social force known only in its effects (Moore, 2013, p.155). It is political, in that it shapes macro relations in society and forms of control in educational processes. Bernstein (2000), and many others (Dewey, 1938; Friere, 1972; Durkheim, 1956), see educational institutions shaped by the social and power relations that underpin society.

Bernstein's pedagogical device presents a theory of instructional and regulative discourses and the relationship between the two (Bernstein, 2000). Instructional discourse is concerned with the transmission and acquisition of specific competencies or skills, namely what is taught and what is assessed in practice; whereas the regulative discourse 'is concerned with the transmission of principles of order, relation and identity' (Bernstein, 2000, p. 32). Bernstein considers this the dominant discourse within the pedagogical relationship. The relationship between the student and midwife will be regulated by three features: the hierarchy, sequence and pace of learning, and criteria for assessment. Each of these can be explicit or implicit.

When the hierarchical rule is explicit, the midwife is in a position of unambiguous super-ordination and student subordination. However, when implicit, the student has more control over their learning. Similarly, explicit or implicit sequencing and criteria affect both the learning and the assessment of learning. When the three features are explicit, a *visible pedagogy* is created (Bernstein, 1977). When the features are implicit, an *invisible pedagogy* is created. Students differ with respect to their understanding and the expectations within visible and invisible pedagogies. Therefore, the device controls who gets what and how.

Using complex explanatory language Bernstein has started a conversation about how these influences affect social action. This is particularly relevant to my study as it enables a discussion of the structure and interaction in midwifery educational relationships. Educational discourses are selectively reproduced at various levels, between agencies, positions, and practices. To explain, the NMC (2009 and 2019) produced the official documents which outline the education of student midwives; this is recontextualised by universities into curricula. Specialised instruction in midwifery is offered in the university setting, and this is extended into the field of practice. Both the field of education and the field of practice may exert influence on the official discourse. When a text, such as the official NMC document, is appropriated by reconstituting agents, the university and practice staff, it undergoes a transformation. It is this transformation, or recontextualisation, that is crucial to the pedagogic device as it acts selectively across available discourses to reinforce or change what counts as legitimate knowledge. The device is located within the space between the NMC, the universities, practice partners, and social beings.

Whether people are aware of the influences of not, they still have the potential to have a profound impact on the individual, as some students will have access to meaning, and others may not. It is this *being social* that structures consciousness and is central to Durkheim's theory; it is also seen in Bernstein's social process of pedagogy, whose work considers macro and micro levels of analysis across educational practices.

Bernstein's theories have been considered at length and used as the conceptual framework for my study because they enable a discussion of the types of knowledge needed for practice and interactions in midwifery education. The implications of distinct types of knowledge and the effects of the relationships on students' learning are important as the midwifery profession needs to understand its pedagogical approaches to increase access to meaning for all students, not just those who 'naturally' understand the education system. This conversation and its application to midwifery education will be continued in each of the findings chapters. The relevance of the relationships and the effect on knowledge production will be explored in the concluding chapter. First, the process of undertaking this research is explained.

2.1.2 Rationale for case study

A case study is useful in studying social life and enabling concepts about social action and structure to be studied (Feagin et al., 1991). Several sources of data are typically used over time to consider the phenomenon holistically. A case study is particularly useful when exploring descriptive questions, such as 'what', or explanatory questions, such as 'how' (Yin, 2009). As the research questions presented in Chapter 1 are descriptive in nature, exploring the phenomenon of grading students' practice, a case study is a suitable methodology. The phenomenon was explored by collecting data in natural settings. For students' experiences, this was in university where they were accustomed to conversing with me as their lecturer, even though at the time I was embodying the role of a researcher. Mentor interviews were mostly conducted in clinical practice, a place where I would usually interact with midwives and discuss student progress.

The strength of the case study design is that it does not specify any specific method for gathering or analysing the data and commonly accommodates quantitative and qualitative elements (Merriam, 1988). My study was broadly qualitative, as I examined participants' experiences in group and individual interviews to answer research questions one, two, and four. However, I also collected the practice grades, which were quantitative, and compared these to the qualitative feedback from mentors. This was to answer research question three. That said, the grades were not seen as fixed objective measures of student practice performance but were understood to be symbolic of the interactions that had occurred between the student and mentor during the placement and agreed in the presence of a lecturer. Therefore, they were subjective interpretations of the students' ability to practice. To understand this subjectivity and reasons for one grade or another, I had to hear the experiences of the participants involved: the students, mentors, and other lecturers.

As a case study researcher, I was the primary instrument for data collection and analysis (Merriam, 1988). With this came ambiguity, what to study, in how much detail, what next, and the issues of sensitivity and integrity of the researcher (Merriam, 1988, p.33). I discuss these in the following sections, but first the case itself.

The case is the experiences of students, mentors, and lecturers when grading students' practice and the meanings attributed to the grade. The case was undertaken at Sanderling University in conjunction with practice partners from three NHS Trusts.

Sanderling University, in partnership with three local NHS Trusts, recruits' applicants to study a BSc (Hons) in Midwifery. Two courses are offered: a three-year direct entry course and a shortened 78-week course for qualified nurses. Each student undertakes theoretical instruction at the university and a range of practice placements in one of the three NHS Trusts. The placements include a consultant-led obstetric unit referred to as the Central Delivery Suite (CDS), midwifery-led birthing unit (MLBU), antenatal and postnatal ward, and community teams. Students spend between 4 and 6 weeks on each placement and return again to each placement during their course. Throughout each placement the student works with a qualified midwife who has undertaken a mentorship course to enable them to teach and assess the student. The requirements of the course and the support in practice are outlined by the regulatory body (NMC, 2009, 2008).

When defining a case, the boundary around places and time periods needs to be stated (Ragin and Becker, 1992). The place is Sanderling University and its partner Trust sites; the time is following the mandatory introduction of grading of midwifery students' practice in the UK (NMC, 2009); the case is the microsocial process of grading practices exploring the experiences of students, mentors, and lecturers when it was introduced and evolved. The microsocial process cannot be explored without considering the macrosocial processes that influence students, mentors, and lecturer's interactions. Thus, a theoretical framework was used to support the analysis of micro and macrosocial practices. The case, therefore, is both empirical and theoretical.

Cases can be unique or particularistic, typical or descriptive, and revelatory or heuristic, depending on the authors' terminology (Yin, 2009; Merriam, 1988). The categories are not mutually exclusive. My case can be considered typical or descriptive in the UK, as midwifery students work with mentors in similar Trusts affiliated to similar universities bound by the same NMC regulations. Therefore, lessons learned from this case may be informative about the experiences of other students, mentors, and lecturers. The case is important for what it reveals about grading midwifery students' practice. However, it is also a unique or particularistic case.

Sanderling University was one of the last UK universities to validate the BSc (Hons) Midwifery curriculum (NMC, 2011). Previously the university had only offered a Diploma in Higher Education in Midwifery. Other UK universities had been delivering graduate-level midwifery education for more than a decade, and many had also been grading students' practice for this length of time (Fisher et al., 2017). Sanderling University was one of the smallest providers of midwifery education in the UK with fewer students, lecturers, and partnership Trusts than many other universities (NMC, 2011). Therefore, the findings may be localised experiences as opposed to national generalisations of grading practices.

To increase the transferability of findings from one local study to a wider population, theories can be used as they play a key role in moving individual concrete experiences to a level of abstract description (Anfara and Mertz, 2006). The process of abstraction includes assigning concepts to distinguish between one event or experience and another; then constructs of related concepts are developed. The relationship between one or several constructs can be explained in propositions. The relationship between the propositions is the theory (Anfara and Mertz, 2006). As already said, the theories used are from Bernstein as his concepts and the relationships between the concepts have been used to interpret the experiences of others in this case and increase their transferability.

2.2 Sampling, participants, and multiple sources of data collection

2.2.1 The midwives

The decision of whom to sample among the midwives was initially open. I wanted to recruit anyone who agreed and who had the experience of grading a student's practice. When posters advertising the study yielded no participants, I purposefully asked individuals to take part, individually in practice and collectively at mentor updates. While this could be seen as undermining the ethical principle of voluntary participation, I was sensitive to this and mentor participation was still voluntary. I knew drawing mentors' attention to the study in a face-to-face encounter could be perceived as a pressure to participate. However, the reactions I received were that none of the mentors had seen the posters; therefore, my convenience recruitment strategy was unsuccessful, and I moved to purposeful sampling. When I explained I was recruiting any mentor who had graded a student's practice, some mentors expressed interest in participating. I ensured the mentors then received the information sheet (Appendix 2) and only followed this up with a date and time to meet when I was confident informed consent had been established (Thomas, 2011).

I had pre-existing relationships with 7 of the 15 mentors. I had been a midwifery lecturer since 2006 and had taught many of the midwives as students. I was particularly mindful of decreasing any expectation that the former students may have felt about participating in my study. I knew I was negotiating a fine line between wanting to include them as valuable sources of information and upholding ethical principles. I explained that the research was separate from my role as lecturer, and they were under no obligation to participate. I made sure every participant knew they could withdraw and did not compel any midwife to organise an interview date.

I recognised the potential for only having participants whom I had a former relationship with as a source of bias, so later in the data collection process I purposely asked mentors who had not trained locally to participate. This ensured the sample was as broad as it could be with only 15 mentors. As the case study progressed, I was aware that I was approaching mentors based on the theories I was developing (Coyne, 1997). I tended to ask mentors whom students said they had developed good relationships with and those able to facilitate learning. Therefore, most midwives were considered 'good' mentors (Hughes and Fraser, 2011; Carolan, 2013; Borrelli, 2014).

In my role as a lecturer, I had a working relationship with most of the mentors as they supported current students. I also had a social relationship with one of the midwives. She was the first midwife interviewed. As a novice researcher, I was more anxious about this interview than any other. The midwife asked if she could be interviewed at my house (near the school her son attended) as it was more convenient for her. Listening to the interview recordings, I discovered that the interviews were different according to the extent to which I engaged, at a personal level, with the interviewee. The more personal the relationship, the more conversational the interview and this led to richer data. With participants I knew less well, the interviews have a feel of formality, and I have the impression their answers were more considered. I was less able to probe these participants. The social interaction between researcher and researched, the assigned roles we embodied, influenced the dialogue and richness of data. Therefore, my anxiety about the first interview and its setting was redundant as it produced one of the most detailed conversations.

Trust 1 was the hardest to recruit participants from; I attribute this to the limited interaction I had with mentors who worked there. I had previously worked as a practising midwife at Trust 3, and I had a role as a link lecturer at Trust 2; I had no specific role at Trust 1. To include staff from this Trust, I agreed for mentors to be interviewed in a group, rather than individually as I had at the other two Trusts. I also had one participant respond electronically to the questions. These issues will be discussed.

The mentors had been employed at the Trusts for variable lengths of time, from 5 to 30 years. Ten of the 15 midwives had been educated locally to certificate or diploma level; three before I started lecturing. Five mentors were purposely chosen, as they were educated elsewhere, these midwives had varying academic qualifications (two had certificates in midwifery, one a diploma, and two were graduates). Eight of the mentors were undertaking post-registration midwifery education, some at degree and others at master's level. This may have contributed to their interest in students' education and/or the research, and enabled them to articulate midwifery knowledge well; hence, they were considered 'good' mentors.

Each mentor was given a participant identifier to depict the order in which they were interviewed, the Trust they worked at and whether they were hospital or community-based. For instance, M1/T3/H was the first mentor to be interviewed; she worked at Trust 3 in the hospital. The decision to differentiate the mentors based on their area of practice stems from the conceptual framework. There was a clear divide between most mentors in how they identified themselves, which was related to where they worked. They tended to identify strongly as community midwives or hospital midwives, except M5 who had recently been appointed to the community, and M6 who had been in the community but was working in the birthing unit. Eight midwives worked in the hospital and seven in the community. The sample of midwives could be considered a 'typical-case selection', since all were regularly mentored students, or an 'ideal-type selection', since most were 'good' mentors (Merriam, 1998, p.50).

2.2.2 Interviews

Interviews are the mainstay of qualitative research and case studies (Yin, 2009; Merriam, 1988). Individual face-to-face semi-structured interviews were conducted with 11 of the 15 mentors. The interviews were audio-recorded, and transcripts created. The rationale for this method of data collection was to enable mentors to discuss their individual experiences of grading student's practice. Interviews are a central data collection method for exploring participant's understandings, opinions, and attitudes (Savin-Baden and Howell Major, 2013). I used semi-structured interviews as I only had one opportunity to hear the participants' narratives and wanted to focus on the interaction. The questions were open-ended to enable discussion (Appendix 3). However, a weakness with this method is that I may not have enabled the participants the opportunity to offer their unique perspectives.

I considered the mentors my colleagues or peers (Platt, 1981); we were jointly involved in the education of student midwives. I did not think there would be a power imbalance between the mentors and myself. However, on reflection, some mentors may have been reluctant to volunteer due to a perceived 'greater' knowledge on my behalf (Platt, 1981). I was a lecturer and may have been seen in a position of authority, especially to the midwives whom I had taught. I did not see myself in a position of power, but I cannot be sure how others saw me. Therefore, I adapted the method of data collection for Trust 1 mentors to enable their participation. Three mentors agreed to a group interview (M10, M11, and M12). The other midwife (M13), who was the most experienced of all mentors, responded electronically to the interview questions, as we could not physically meet due to competing work patterns.

The interviews occurred in two phases, the pilot phase in June 2011 to test the questions and core phase from January–September 2013. The interview schedule consisted of ten questions relating to mentors' experiences of grading: the process and tool (Appendix 3). One change was made to the questions for the core phase: I included one further 'how' question on teaching and learning (Appendix 3, version 2, question 3). Participant information sheets and consent forms were discussed and signed prior to beginning and recording the interviews (Appendix 2 and 4).

All except one of the interviews were undertaken in the workplace. This included hospital clinical rooms, coffee and office spaces, community children's centres, and an education centre room. While it was possible to book a private space in the education centre, this was not possible in the hospital; therefore, the space chosen was whatever was available. Eight mentor interviews were conducted during their working day (M2, M3, M4, M6, M8, M9, M14 and M15); this affected the time available, and these interviews were the shortest. Some of the interviews were interrupted briefly, sometimes because the midwife was holding the drug cupboard keys, and sometimes she was asked to verify something. When interruptions occurred, we stopped talking, to keep confidentiality, and continued once the room was private again.

As the study progressed, I tried to conduct the interviews slightly away from the clinical environment, in the coffee room, for example, to reduce interruptions. However, we met other disturbances there. When this happened, we waited for the other person to leave the room and continued our interview in private. Interruptions would happen when I visited mentors and students in practice too, and this seemed to add to the authenticity of the conversations. It also highlighted how little time and space is available for mentors and students to discuss students' performance privately.

The interviews were as naturalistic as possible, recognising that participants may withhold or over emphasise ideas and information to fit with their projected identity (Lambert and Loiselle, 2008). An ethical dilemma in research is the imbalance of power between the researcher and research participant (Trimmer, 2016). Recognising this, I reassured mentors that they were the experts in practice, not me, to reduce any perceived structural imbalance. While there were no specific relational problems during the interviews, a few of the mentors gave brief answers to the questions posed (Roulston, 2014). As a novice researcher, initially

I did not manage to probe the mentor for further ideas, but as I relaxed and became more confident in the process a more conversational dialogue ensued.

Three individual mentors (M1, M5, M7) and the group interview (M10, M11 and M12) were conducted outside the midwives paid employment time. The group interview lasted 58 minutes, as there were more opinions to hear and discussions; M5, similarly, lasted 53 minutes. M7's interview was shorter, although it was not in work time, she was scheduled to commence her shift 30 minutes after our appointment time. I was particularly mindful that I was taking up mentors' time and only asked for 30 minutes even though the participant information sheet specified up to 1 hour. With hindsight, I could have asked for longer although I recognise this as an ethical tension as I was either asking mentors to make time in their busy working day or their personal life to contribute to the research.

Table 2.1 Summary of mentor interview date, place, commitment to work, and time

Date	Place	Participant/work commitment	Time in minutes
Pilot phase			
20 June 2011	My house	M1/T3/H – off duty	18
20 June 2011	Trust 3 Ward office	M2/T3/H – on duty	10
20 June 2011	Trust 3 Ward office	M3/T3/H – on duty	10
21 June 2011	Trust 3 CDS clinical room	M4/T3/C – on duty	17
Core phase			
30 January 2013	Trust 2 Education centre room	M5/T2/C – off duty	53
20 February 2013	Trust 2 MLBU clinical room	M6/T2/H+C – on duty	44
5 March 2013	Trust 2 CDS clinical room	M7/T2/H – off duty	25
12 March 2013	Trust 3 Children's centre clinical room	M8/T3/C – on duty	22
12 March 2013	Trust 3 Children's centre clinical room	M9/T3/C – on duty	31
3 June 2013	Trust 1 CDS clinical room	M10/T1/H and M11/T1/H and M12/T1/C – all off duty	58
1 September 2013	Virtual (email)	M13/T1/C – unknown	unknown
10 September 2013	CDS staff room Trust 2	M14/T2/H – on duty	18
10 September 2013	CDS staff room Trust 2	M15/T2/H – on duty	29
Total			5 hours 35 minutes

2.2.3 The students

By contrast, the students were entirely self-selected. I was particularly careful that no student felt excluded or favoured; therefore, all students in each year were invited. The 2009, 2011, and 2012 cohorts represent the largest numbers; these are students on the three-year course (see Table 2.2). Between 62–76% of the students in these cohorts volunteered. The 2012 and 2013 shortened course cohorts consisted of six students, respectively, so most of these students volunteered too (83–100%). The 2010 three-year cohort was least represented due to timing with ethical approval; by the time I had approval for the core phase of data collection this cohort of students had qualified (n=11). Therefore, it was harder to recruit from this cohort. The high number of students per cohort reduced the bias of self-selected groups.

I had built a relationship with all the students over time before the research began. They knew me as a lecturer, module leader for research, and I was the personal tutor for many students at Trust 2. The students were, therefore, familiar with my presence in the university and witnessed my ordinary working life. A few students I knew less well; however, I was aware in the group interviews they seemed to trust me with their experiences.

2.2.4 Group interviews

The rationale for using group interviews with the students was to counterbalance the potential power differential between myself as their lecturer, although I was a researcher at the time, and the students, and to hear different experiences (Liamputtong, 2011). Individual interviews may have felt too intense for the students as their personal experience and grade would have been discussed. Focus groups are a key approach where interpretative and pedagogical issues are examined, especially when considering symbolic interactionism or critical pedagogical practice (Liamputtong, 2011). As this study was about understanding pedagogical practice and interactions, I considered it the best method to collect data from the students. Some authors differentiate between a group interview and a focus group (Thomas, 2011) others do not (Merriam, 1988). In the group interview, the researcher takes the lead with the questioning, in the focus group

Table 2.2 Student sample and percentage of cohort

Cohort	Number of students	Number/cohort size=percentage
2009 (3 year)	11 students, (pilot)	11/16=68%
2010 (3 year)	2 students	2/11=18%
2011 (3 year)	11 students	11/17=62%
2012 (3 year)	16 students	16/21=76%
2012S (shortened)	5 students	5/6=83%
2013S (shortened)	6 students	6/6=100%
51 students in total		

Table 2.3 Summary of student group interviews, dates, times, and transcription length

Date	Groups	Number of participants	Time in minutes
Pilot phase			
10 June 2011	G1	4	28
10 June 2011	G2	4	29
10 June 2011	G3	3	6
Core phase			
28 November 2012	G4S (shortened)	5	44
3 December 2012	G5	6	59
10 December 12	G6	5	59
16 May 2013	G7	5	46
16 May 2013	G8	5	67
16 May 2013	G9	6	61
26 June 2013	G10	2	48
26 September 2013	G11S (shortened)	6	47
Total		51	8 hours 14 minutes

the researcher facilitates or moderates (Thomas, 2011). As I took the lead by asking questions, to hearing multiple experiences, this research uses the term 'group interview'.

The participant information sheet and consent forms were distributed and signed prior to audio recording the discussions (Appendix 2 and 4). All the group interviews were conducted in the university buildings. As FG10 participants had already qualified, they came in on their day off work; however, all other interviews were within the university's scheduled teaching day at break times (See Table 2.3). All the groups were homogenous in that they had students from just one cohort; this is considered a necessity by some authors, as it generates better data with groups that know each other (McLafferty, 2004). I did not choose the homogenous approach for methodological reasons; it was a practical decision as only one cohort of students tended to be in university at a time.

To maximise discussion, the students suggested that they could get into groups that were mixed across the three Trusts. I did not try to organise this as I wanted all students to feel comfortable in front of their peers, as disclosure in front of other participants is a criticism of focus groups (Liamputtong, 2011). With the larger three-year student cohorts where there are dynamics unknown to the researcher, I felt it particularly important students organised whose group they were in.

The group interviews used a semi-structured approach based on the participants' experiences and grading processes (Appendix 3). Staff sickness on the day of the pilot study meant I needed to facilitate teaching and was not free to facilitate the group interviews. I asked the students whether they wanted to cancel the interviews and reconvene or conduct the group interview independently using the interview questions. They decided to undertake unfacilitated group interviews. While this approach worked well in illuminating some discussions, which may not have occurred had I been present, some ideas expressed would have benefitted from further clarification. Additionally, the third group interview recording was stopped at 6 minutes, this may have been intentional or accidental, but I do not know which.

For the core group interviews, I was present and followed up on aspects of the discussions I did not fully understand, and I noticed who spoke, their emotions, and when they interrupted or supported others. The students were incredibly open; they even offered unexpected responses about my colleagues, which I had not considered in the first ethical approval process (McConnell-Henry et al., 2010). I had the sense that students trusted me. The recordings appear rich, personal, and spontaneous. However, because students interrupted and reminded each other of events, the conversations, at times, were fragmented.

Students are identified by the number in which they contributed, Trust and group (S1/T2/G1).

2.2.5 The lecturers

The lecturers were invited to a group discussion. This discussion was planned to occur as late in the data collection process as possible, to capture the collective experiences of the grading process and tripartite meetings we had participated in. All five lecturers agreed to participate. The rationale for this group discussion was to hear my peers' experiences of grading but also for research credibility and triangulation of findings (Houghton et al., 2013). My peers had attended an equal number of student–mentor grading meetings, understood the curriculum, and were part of its delivery and student support; it was essential to hear how their experiences and thoughts differed or resonated with my own, the mentors', and the students'.

The discussion was undertaken during a lunch break when all lecturers were available; it lasted 55 minutes. The group discussions corroborated many of the students' experiences. In this way, triangulation occurred.

Listening to the three sources of interview data collected, differences are noted between the individual and group recordings. Individual interviews tended to have longer passages of uninterrupted talk from the participants, and their focus was maintained. Whereas, group interviews tended to produce more fractured talk. However, the student data was particularly rich in detail and emotion, this may be because the students often discussed their practice experiences, and the 'talk' was more spontaneous. It may also be that the student group interviews were productive because I was used to facilitating group discussions with these participants in my teaching role. The skill I had developed as a lecturer was brought to the research context. In all, the interviews produced a set of individual accounts through interactions with me, or in the case of the group interviews through exchanges and interactions with peers and myself. These accounts, collectively, were the basis of the case study.

2.2.6 Documentary data

To complement the interview data and utilise multiple sources, documentary data was included in this case study. Documents are convenient sources of evidence (Merriam, 1988). A range of documents were collected electronically, such as all 124 student practice grades from 2010 to 2015, 12 individual student action plans, and meeting minutes. These were stored on a password-protected computer. Hard copies of 26 student Practice Assessment Documents (PADs) were also collected once students had completed their education. The PADs would be considered a convenience sample: some were available to the researcher because they had not been collected by the students; others were offered to the researcher. The sample of PADs was from students on both courses and different cohorts (2009S, 2009, 2010S, 2010, 2011, and 2012).

Permission to use the PADs was given from the university. However, students gave implicit permission when they handed their PAD to me for the study too. These were anonymised. If the student had taken part in the group interviews, this identification code was used, if not a new code was given. This enabled cross-referencing between the student comments and the documentary data in some cases, but not others.

Documents are usually produced for reasons other than research; thus, information within them may not fit the research focus. This was certainly the case with my collection of documents. Some of the data collected, such as Course Committee minutes, Student Course Handbooks, curriculum development evidence, National Student Survey results, and midwifery team meeting minutes were not used. However, other data such as students' practice grades, a sample of PADs and student action plans enabled a deeper focus on grading practices.

A limitation of using documentary evidence is that data is sometimes missing (Merriam, 1988); this was the case with two students' PADs. These PADs did not record all the students' learning, one had transferred into the university, the other had lost her PAD, and the replacement had no early entries.

2.3 Ethical approval

As a novice researcher, I wanted to conduct a pilot study to gain research interview experience and test my interview questions. Gaining access from the two universities, the one I was studying at and one I worked at and collected data from, was straightforward. However, gaining access to the hospitals was a long, complex, and frustrating process. Approval for the pilot study (reference 10/H0310/45) took 13 months, with one of three NHS sites declining my request for access (Appendix 5).

My intention was to interview one or two midwives from each Trust; in the end, I had four from Trust 3. Reflecting on the pilot study data, I recognised I needed to ask more 'how' questions to mentors. I had asked about assessing students without asking how the mentors facilitated learning or taught the students. I, therefore, amended the questions for the core phase (Appendix 3).

The second round of ethical approval for the core study was equally time-consuming (11 months). Final clearance was gained on 22 April 2013. This time I had access to all three NHS sites (Appendix 5).

2.3.1 *Ethical considerations, identity, relationships, and authority*

Researching in one's workplace was a complex process (Coghlan and Brannick, 2009). Being an insider-researcher was an advantage as I had valuable knowledge about midwifery, many of the participants, the educational cultures under study, and the informal structures in the organisations. However, it was also a disadvantage as I was part of the organisation and its culture. As an insider, when interviewing staff and students I understood what they were saying and therefore did not probe as much as I might have done had I been an outsider, to fully explore what 'things' meant. The boundaries between insider and outsider were also lower than expected at times, with students and mentors disclosing information I would not usually have known (Williams, 2010). Thus, the dual responsibility of being a lecturer and researcher was hard to balance and caused ethical considerations (Coghlan and Brannick, 2009).

I did not fully understand the nature of qualitative research *sui generis* (Williams, 2010). When participants disclosed personal subjective experiences, I understood the meaning of 'guilty knowledge' (ibid, p.256). In qualitative case studies, according to Merriam (1988), the ethical dilemmas are more likely to emerge at the data collection and dissemination of findings phase. I experienced several ethical dilemmas during data collection, including recruiting mentors, as discussed earlier. I am aware that my interpretation of some of the student's narratives or PAD entries might not be their interpretation and could be upsetting, so I am mindful of this when disseminating my findings. When students and mentors told me my peers had missed or forgotten meetings or 'interfered' in the grading process I worried about what to do with the information. I had promised the participants confidentiality (except if there had been a breach of the NMC Code) and knew this must be respected.

I considered explaining to my peers the effect their behaviour had on the students so they would not cause potential distress to other students but knew I could not do this. I wondered how I would handle this sensitive data in the narrative case. Disseminating potentially damaging reports of colleagues has political and professional ramifications. Once the lecturers disclosed these experiences in the group discussion, and I knew they had worried about whether they should or should not have influenced the grading process, I felt slightly less guilty knowing what happened. However, I still have a duty to show where power lies in grading students' performance.

I wondered whether asking the students about their experiences of grading and negotiating their grades made them more aware of their power in this process. Some had already noticed the weaknesses in the system and the potential to negotiate which mentor they worked with or who graded their practice. This may have empowered others to negotiate a more lenient mentor to influence the grading process. Most of the time, I do not believe this happened. Those students who understood how the system worked often had the authority to alter their chance of a positive grading outcome. This is addressed in more detail in Chapter 4. Those who could not alter their access to learning opportunities or grade were not unaware of how mentorship or grading worked; they often had a poor mentor-student relationship which afforded no opportunity for negotiation.

I was most concerned about a student who disclosed reports of bullying behaviour from mentors in practice. She had already reported these instances, so I was able to hear her experiences, offer her support and record them in the case study without following up on the allegation. Conversely, I was slightly disappointed when a student was too upset to join the group interview and discuss her practice experiences due to her low grade. I sat and listened to her experience, half wishing she had said it all 'on the tape', as it was valuable data lost, but my role at that time was as a lecturer and not a researcher.

As the newest and only part-time member of the midwifery team when I started this research, I worried about my status within the team and whether my research was affecting the grading practices at Sanderling University. The midwifery team implemented changes to the validated grading tool as several challenges to the new assessment process were noted. Unfortunately, the first change increased the student practice grades, so a further amendment to the grading tool was made. The changes and effects of these are evident in the data collected from both students and mentors. However, at the time, I wondered whether I was driving the assessment changes as I was noticing the issues, and there might have been fewer changes had I not been researching the assessment process.

Over time, the lecturing team changed. I became full-time, was promoted, and early drafts of this work (Chenery-Morris, 2014, 2015) and research with others (Fisher et al., 2017, 2018) were published. I worried less about being a junior member of the team and my novice researcher status. However, some of my achievements came at a time when other members of the team had significant stress and poor health, which affected their well-being and work performance. During the data collection process, I paid attention to being empathetic with my colleagues and participants, not just because it is an ethical principle in research to uphold (Patton, 2002), but it is a professional responsibility and social imperative.

At the outset of this case study, I assumed that all sources of data had equal weight. However, as the case study developed, I realised I was drawing on more references to the students' experiences than the mentors or lecturers. In part, this was because I had more student data, but also the students could explain how grading made them feel and had specific examples of their experiences. Mentors and lecturers, alternatively, tended to talk more generally about their role. There were fewer consequences for the mentors or lecturers if they awarded a student a low practice grade. Whereas the students articulated strong emotional responses related to their practice experiences and grading. Therefore, there is more emphasis on the students' voices than the mentors or lecturers. This causes an ethical concern as participants may expect more of their 'side' presented in this work, and it might not be there, despite having found time for the interviews. All perspectives were heard; however, the voice of the students has taken centre stage, supported, or refuted by the other respondents. This is because the structural and interactional processes are most clear in their discussions. Grading meant more to them, so they seemed to notice and explain these issues.

2.3.2 Ethical challenges

As a lecturer and researcher in the university and partnership Trusts where the study took place, it was important for me to consider my position as an insider and outsider. Indeed, any interpretive approach should reflect upon the role of the researcher as the primary instrument of data collection (Merriam, 1988). At all times, I tried to reduce power differences to encourage disclosure and authenticity between myself and the participants (Karniele-Miller et al., 2009). However, in doing so, I faced some ethical tensions.

In recruiting participants, I explained why I was undertaking the research in the participant information letter, but purposely withheld my view that grading practice was complex, subjective, and that I was not convinced every student who received a first warranted one. However, when asked directly during data collection I answered honestly. In one student group interview this led to a good discussion about the difference between theoretical and practice assessment criteria.

When a participant and I reflected upon our discussions, I had inadvertently left the audio recorder on but did not realise this until I listened back to the recording the following day. The reflections were more illuminating than the formal recording had been, yet I knew I could not use this as data. The participant had not consented to it, and it was not part of her chosen responses. Our post-interview discussions had been more in-depth because I had opened up more when I thought the recording had stopped, and so did the participant. I considered starting subsequent interviews with an informal chat about grading, but then worried this would influence what participants said. The tension between maximising access to participants' real experiences and feelings and building a sense of rapport and equal relationship between us was delicate. I managed this better with some participants than others.

Holding difficult knowledge about others was also a challenge that had the potential to affect the quality of the data interpretation. For instance, while most of the mentors were considered good by students, I had heard stories and instances about ineffective mentoring about one or two participants. This had the potential to lead me to less positive interpretations of their experiences. However, I had to overcome this as all the participants may have given socially desirable responses and I had no way of knowing whose account was more valid than another's, so I had to treat all as equally valid. I offered participants the opportunity to review their transcripts and to alter any misinterpretations; however, only one accepted. The mentor who reviewed her transcript commented upon the number of conversational fillers (umm and err), they seemed to prompt worry over how she was represented. Following this, I removed all conversational fillers from the transcripts and vignettes used in this work.

In considering these tensions, I feel I have upheld the ethical guidelines. I did not distort the meaning of the participants' voices. The participants' own language is presented in vignettes prior to my interpretation. I maintained the anonymity of the participants through participant identifiers. I have used the female pronoun for the one male midwifery student to preserve his anonymity and abstracted some of the concerns regarding students who were underperforming. In this way, I have reduced the potential for participants to be identified by others who may know them. However, there is the potential that some of the individuals may recognise their own experiences. Managing the tension between holding difficult knowledge and representing an authentic case has been pervasive. Ultimately, I tried to uphold the ethical principle of non-maleficence.

2.4 Data analysis strategy

Using a qualitative case study approach meant that data was collected and analysed simultaneously. The process of data collection and analysis was recursive. I listened frequently to the audio recordings, but a third party transcribed the data verbatim. While this may distance the researcher from the primary data, each transcript was checked for accuracy and amendments were made when related to specific midwifery terminology, such as cinto instead of synto(cinon). Only the words or utterances were transcribed not the tone, pacing, timing, or pauses. This decision impacted upon the interpretation of the data as participant hesitation or certainty could have been included in the analysis. However, as human interaction is so complex, and the process of transcription is essentially one of data reduction, the added information may have made the usability of the transcripts more difficult, and it was the content of the conversations I initially needed rather than the interactions themselves. That said, as the analysis progressed, I found myself drawn to discourse analysis of the speech and text patterns.

Discourse analysis is not a specific method but a way of analysing language, whether written, spoken, or signed (Savin-Baden and Howell Major, 2013). It is often used in case studies and provides insights into human communication and interaction (Savin-Baden and Howell Major, 2013). As the discourse, the communication in midwifery, was central to my study, it seemed relevant to explore how participants understood society and human behaviour. Discourse analysis has grown in the study of the sociology of knowledge and interactionism (Somekh and Lewin, 2011), both elements of my research; however, it was a small part of the analysis strategy.

The main analysis strategy started with coding through notes or memos on the transcripts to record my emerging ideas (Merriam, 1988; Silverman, 2011). I then developed codes to describe and analyse the transcripts. The codes included behaviours, patterns, relationships, interactions, and consequences heard from the recordings and read in the transcripts (Savin-Baden and Howell Major, 2013).

Initially, the codes were open codes, labels such as time, professionalism, communication with women, and confidence were applied to the data (Appendix 9). The second phase of coding was axial. These codes were informed by Bernstein's concepts of classification, framing, hierarchy, sequencing and pacing, and criteria. The axial codes enabled me to make connections between the categories (Appendix 9). Even though data was collected in two phases; pilot and core, once data collection was completed, the analysis intensified and considered both phases together as the whole case rather than separate parts.

Analysis of the grades was easy: I tabulated them and could count frequencies and generate descriptive statistics from this. Analysis of the PAD and action plan documents was more difficult. It began with questions I had about how the document was used, how often it was used, and what individual comments meant. The PAD documents contained handwritten feedback from mentors to students on their performance for every placement in their course and the practice grades. Action plans were developed if a student was underperforming in a placement area. Each year a few students are on action plans, some students succeed and pass their placement, a few leave the course, and a small number are referred in practice. Thus, the action plans were created, usually by lecturers after a discussion with the mentor and student, to signify to underperforming students the areas of practice they needed to develop. These were reviewed on a weekly or fortnightly basis and updated.

Two types of analysis were used: content and discourse. Content analysis of the PADs included counting how many placements each student had, whether their progress had been discussed at the planned times (initial, mid-point and end-point of the placement), how similar the student's self-assessed grade and mentor's grade were, and whether the mentor's written comments matched the grade awarded; this is presented in Chapter 5. Content of the action plans included categorising reasons for student underperformance and determining themes from this, as presented in Chapter 6. A discourse analysis of the language and styles used within the PADs was also undertaken. The PADs represented a convention in that mentors would presumably have verbally explained to the students' their practice strengths and weaknesses and then written a synopsis of their discussion in the document.

From the content analysis, I observed that some students wrote their own feedback; usually, this was the mid-point feedback rather than end-point feedback. This could be interpreted to mean the mid-point interview is not as important as the summative evaluation, even though pedagogically, it could be argued, it is more important. I analysed whether mentors elevated students' practice grades or reduced them and discuss this in Chapter 5. The discourse analysis enabled an interpretation of the symbols used within the mentor's feedback, such as smiley faces, exclamation marks, and underlining. These features, and the words used, were interpreted to ascertain negotiation of power, and meaning and relationships between students and mentors. Students' comments who had participated in the group interview were cross-referenced to the action plans and PADs to see if there was a relationship between the forms of evidence.

Key stages and analytical decisions included:

1. Ending data collection. By the time I had analysed the entire interview data, I was confident that no new themes were emerging, so theoretical saturation had occurred (Guest et al., 2006). McLafferty (2004) suggests that data generated after ten focus groups is usually redundant; similarly 12 participants are likely to be sufficient for individual interviews (Guest et al., 2006). As I had more than both these authors suggest, I was confident I had enough qualitative data.

2. The next step was to organise the case study database (Yin, 2009). I compiled a chronological account of events which could be significant. This included the dates of the interviews and changes to the grading tools to see if there were observations or questions I needed to follow up.

3. I now recognise I had far more data than I needed; thus, I needed to exclude some data from the case study. Initially, this was a difficult decision for me because I could see some relevance to much of the documentary data I had collected. However, over time I narrowed the focus of the study and excluded midwifery team meeting minutes and other forms of documentary data from the analysis.

4. The memos, coupled with the evidence from the literature review, initiated quantitative ideas for analysis, such as what is the compliance with the clinical meeting reviews documented in the PAD? How much variation is there between students regarding the number of placements and the timeliness of feedback? The generation of descriptive statistics then lead to qualitative questioning, such as what potential effect does this have on students' learning and on the evaluation of that? Similarly, when students said mentors frequently elevated their practice grade, the PADs were examined to see how often and the amount the grade was raised. Thus, the analysis included finding data to support generalisations made during the interviews and relationships between concepts (Merriam, 1988, p.69).

5. The balance between empirical data description and application of the theoretical framework was omnipresent. Initially, open coding undertaken in NVivo 10 was inductive, I asked myself 'what does this student or mentor's experience mean' can a label be applied to its content. This open coding was a labour-intensive process undertaken over several months at the weekends. I was hesitant about 'making mistakes'; however, once axial coding, using Bernstein's educational transmission codes was applied to the data, I became more confident with the analysis process (Appendix 9). The relationship between the participants' experiences and educational transmission process became clearer and could be articulated. For instance, students described experiences where midwives were unprofessional in their manner. Bernstein's theory enabled 'the manner' of the midwife to be understood and described in relation to their status relative to the student. Due to the hierarchy between the midwife and student, the student was unable to comment in clinical practice about a midwife's behaviour; however, the student

usually observed this, and it affected the criteria by which she then evaluated the midwife's performance and this in turn influenced whether the midwife's evaluation of the student was considered valid or not. Bernstein's theory also framed the three main findings chapters: what counts as valid practice knowledge, the transmission of knowledge in clinical practice, and the evaluation of learning.

6. Initially, I analysed the quantitative and qualitative data from the students on the three-year course separately from the 78-week course, looking for differences between them. While there are some differences, explained in the findings, I was surprised about how many similarities there were in their practice grades and experiences. Thus, most of the time, I do not separate or differentiate between the students.

7. While codes and themes were important in the analysis, I found myself drawn to analysing the discourse of participants. What did it mean when students or mentors used specific words? There is, therefore, an element of discourse analysis in the research.

I appreciate the analysis strategy may appear eclectic; however, it was important to analyse the data from several perspectives to see if this illuminated innovative ideas. While Bernstein's (2000) theory was immensely helpful in explaining the significance of my findings, I am aware, in using his theory, I may have inadvertently missed some important inductive finding. However, I believe this research can contribute to the body of knowledge on grading students' practice. All students have the potential to be midwives, they are selected through a rigorous process, yet not all students reach their potential. Bernstein's theory has enabled the inequality in access to knowledge to be considered to potentially improve midwifery education, so all students have equal opportunity to practise midwifery.

In summary of the above discussion, a qualitative case approach was undertaken to investigate grading students' practice. The aim was to explore how grading influences and affects midwifery students' mentors and lecturers' relationships, identity, and authority. Multiple methods were used to collect data from various sources. These included a semi-structured approach for individual and group interviews with mentors, students, and lecturers. Documentary analysis included students' grades, Practice Assessment Documents and underperforming student action plans. The data was analysed with a combination of computer-assisted tools and manually using open and axial coding based on Bernstein's theories, which combine structure and interaction. The limitations of the case study method have been addressed by the closeness of the researcher to the research, triangulation of the multiple sources, data saturation, and member and peer checking.

Bibliography

Anfara, V. A. & Mertz, N. T., (2006). *Theoretical Frameworks for Qualitative Research*. London: SAGE Ltd.

Atkinson, P., (1985). *Language, Structure and Reproduction An Introduction to the Sociology of Basil Bernstein*. Abingdon: Routledge.

Atkinson, P. & Housley, W., (2003). *Interactionism*. London: SAGE Ltd.

Begley, C., (2001). 'Knowing your place': Student midwives' views of relationships in midwifery in Ireland. *Midwifery*, 17(3), pp. 222–233.

Begley, C., (2002). Great fleas have little fleas: Irish student midwives' views of the hierarchy in midwifery. *Journal of Advanced Nursing*, 38(3), pp. 310–317.

Benner, P., (2001). *From Novice to Expert Excellence and Power in Clinical Nursing Practice*. London: Prentice-Hall International (UK) Limited.

Bernstein, B., (1977). *Class, Codes and Control Volume III*. 2nd ed. London: Routledge.

Bernstein, B., (1990). *Class, Codes and Control Volume VI The Structuring of Pedagogic Discourse*. London: Routledge Taylor and Francis Group.

Bernstein, B., (2000). *Pedagogy, Symbolic Control and Identity Theory, Research, Critique*. 2nd ed. Oxford: s.n.

Borrelli, S. E., (2014). What is a good midwife? Insights from the literature. *Midwifery*, 30(1), pp. 3–10.

Carolan, M., (2013). 'A good midwife stands out': 3rd year midwifery students' views. *Midwifery*, 29(2), pp. 115–121.

Carper, B., (1978). Fundamental patterns of knowing in nursing. *Advances in Nursing Science*, 1(1), pp. 13–23.

Chenery-Morris, S., (2014). Exploring student and mentors experiences of grading midwifery practice, *Evidence-Based Practice*, 12(2), pp. 101–106.

Chenery-Morris, S., (2015). The importance of continuity of mentorship in pre-registration midwifery education, *Evidence Based Midwifery*, 13(2), pp.47–53.

Christiensen, P. & James, A., (2008). *Research with Children: Perspective and Practices*. 2nd ed. Oxon: Routledge.

Coghlan, D. & Brannick, T., (2009). *Doing Action Research in Your own Organisation*. Abingdon: Routledge.

Collins, R., (2000). *The Sociology of Philosophies; A Global Theory of Intellectual Change*. Cambridge, MA: Harvard University Press.

Coyne, I., (1997). Sampling in qualitative research: Purposeful and theoretical sampling; merging or clear boundaries?. *Journal of Advanced Nursing*, 26, pp. 623–630.

Danzig, A., (1995). Applications and distortions of Basil Bernstein's code theory. In: A. Sandovik, ed. *Knowledge and Pedagogy: The Sociology of Basil Bernstein*. Norwood, NJ: Ablex Publishing.

Deery, R., (2005). An action-research study exploring midwives' support needs and the affect of group clinical supervision. *Midwifery*, 21(2), pp. 161–176.

Denzin, N., (2001). *Interpretive Interactionism*. London: Sage Publications.

Dewey, J., (1938). *Experience and Education*. New York: Collier Books.

Durkheim, E., (1956). *Education and Sociology*. Toronto: The Free Press.

Eraut, M., (1994). *Developing Professional Knowledge and Competence*. London: Falmer Press.

Feagin, J., Orum, A. & Sjoberg, G., (1991). *A Case for the Case Study*. Chapel Hill: University of North Carolina Press.

Fenwick, J., Hammond, A., Raymond, J., Smith, R., Gray, J., Foureue, M. & Symon, A., (2012). Surviving, not thriving: A qualitative study of newly qualified midwives' experience of their transition to practice. *Journal of Clinical Nursing*, 21(13–14), pp. 2054–2063.

Fisher, M., Bower, H., Chenery-Morris, S., Jackson, J. & Way, S., (2017). A scoping study to explore the application and impact of grading practice in pre-registration midwifery programmes across the United Kingdom. *Nurse Education in Practice*, 24, pp. 99–105.

Fisher, M., Bower, H., Chenery-Morris, S., Jackson, J. & Way, S., (2018). National survey: Developing a common approach to grading of practice in pre-registration midwifery. *Nurse Education in Practice*.

Frandji, D. & Vitale, P., (2011). *Knowledge, Pedagogy and Society International Perspectives on Basil Bernstein's Sociology of Education*. Abingdon: Routledge.

Friere, P., (1972). *Pedagogy of the Oppressed*. Harmondsworth: Penguin Books.

Gee, J. P., 2000. Identity as an analytical lens for research in education. *Review of Research in Education*, 25, pp. 99–125.

Guest, G., Bunce, A. & Johnson, L., (2006). How many interviews are enough? An experiment with data saturation and variability. *Field Methods*, 18(1), pp. 59–82.

Harker, R. & May, A., (1993). Code and habitus: Comparing the accounts of Bernstein and Bordieu. *British Journal of Sociology of Education (London)*, 14(2), pp. 169–178.

Houghton, C., Casey, D., Shaw, D. & Murphy, K., (2013). Rigour in qualitative case-study research. *Nurse Researcher*, 20(4), pp. 12–17.

Hughes, A. J. & Fraser, D. M., (2011). There are guiding hands and there are controlling hands': Student midwives experience of mentorship in the UK. *Midwifery*, 27(4), pp. 477–483.

Hunter, B., (2005). Conflicting ideologies as a source of emotion in midwifery. *Midwifery*, 21(3), pp. 253–266.

Karniele-Miller, O., Strier, R. & Pessach, L., (2009). Power relations in qualitative research. *Qualitative Health Research*, 19(2), pp. 279–289.

King, R., (1976). Bernstein's sociology of the school: Some propositions tested. *British Journal of Sociology (London)*, 27(4), pp. 430–443.

Lambert, S. D. & Loiselle, C. G., (2008). Combining individual interviews and focus groups to enhance data richness. *Journal of Advanced Nursing*, 62(2), pp. 228–237.

Liamputtong, P., (2011). *Focus Group Methodology*. London: SAGE Publishing.

McConnell-Henry, T., James, A., Chapman, Y. & Francis, K., (2010). Researching with people you know: Issues in interviewing. *Contemporary Nurse: A Journal for the Australian Nursing Profession*, 34(1), pp. 2–9.

McLafferty, I., (2004). Focus group interviews as a data collecting strategy. *Journal of Advanced Nursing*, 48(2), pp. 187–194.

Merriam, S., (1988). *Case Study Research in Education A Qualitative Approach*. San Francisco: Jossey-Bass Publishers.

Moore, R., (2013). *Basil Bernstein The Thinker and the Field*. Abingdon: Routledge.

Muller, J., (2006). On the shoulders of giants: Verticality of knowledge and the school curriculum. In: R. Moore, M. Arnot, J. Beck & H. Daniels, eds. *Knowledge, Power and Educational Reform: Applying the Sociology of Basil Bernstein*. London: Routledge, pp. 11–27.

Muller, J., Davies, B. & Morais, A., (2004). *Reading Bernstein, Researching Bernstein*. London: Routledge Farmer.

NMC, (2008). *Standards to Support Learning and Assessment in Practice*. London: Nursing and Midwifery Council.

NMC, (2009). *Standards for Pre-Registration Midwifery Education*. London: Nursing and Midwifery Council.

NMC, (2011). *MINT (Midwives IN Teaching) Final Report*. London: Nursing and Midwifery Council.

NMC, (2019). *Standards of Proficiency for Midwives*. London: Nursing and Midwifery Council.

Patton, M., (2002). *Qualitative Research and Evaluation Methods*. Thousand Oaks, CA: SAGE.

Pickering, W. S. F., (2000). *Durkheim and Representations*. London: Routledge.

Platt, J., (1981). On interviewing one's peers. *British Journal of Sociology*, 32(1), pp. 75–91.

Ragin, C. & Becker, H., (1992). *What is a Case? Exploring the Foundations of Social Inquiry.* Cambridge: Cambridge University Press.

Rosen, H., (1972). *Language and Class: A Critical Look at the Theories of Basil Bernstein.* Bristol: Falling Wall Press.

Roulston, K., (2014). Interactional problems in research interviews. *Qualitative Research*, 14(3), pp. 277–293.

Sandovnik, A. R., (1995). *Knowledge and Pedagogy: The Sociology of Basil Bernstein.* New Jersey: Ablex Publishing Corporation.

Savin-Baden, M. & Howell Major, C., (2013). *Qualitative Research the Essential Guide to Theory and Practice.* Abingdon: Routledge.

Silverman, D., (2011). *Interpreting Qualitative Data.* 4th ed. London: SAGE Ltd.

Somekh, B. & Lewin, C., (2011). *Theory and Methods in Social Research.* 2nd ed. London: SAGE Ltd.

Thomas, G., (2011). *How to Do Your Case Study a Guide for Students and Researchers.* London: SAGE Publishing Ltd.

Trimmer, K., (2016). *Political Pressures on Educational and Social Research International Perspectives.* Oxon: Routledge.

van Vuuren, M. & Westerhof, G. J., (2015). Identity as 'knowing your place': The narrative construction of space in a healthcare profession. *Journal of Health Psychology*, 20(3), pp. 326–337.

Williams, K., (2010). Guilty knowledge the (im)possibility of ethical security in social science research. In: P. Thomson, and M. Walker, eds. *The Routledge Doctoral Student's Companion.* Oxon: Routledge, pp. 256–269.

Yin, R., (2009). *Case Study Research Designs and Methods.* London: SAGE Ltd.

3 What counts as valid practice knowledge?

This chapter is the first of three chapters that report the project's findings, drawing on Bernstein's theorisation of formal educational knowledge. Early in the data analysis, the importance of practice for students was noted. Practice had higher status relative to theoretical knowledge. However, when asked what encompassed effective midwifery practice, students and mentors alike had difficulty articulating this practice knowledge. During the analysis, three forms of practice knowledge were noted as being discussed often by the students and mentors. These were communication and interpersonal skills, specific clinical skills, and evidence to inform practice. These types of practice knowledge are then explored using Bernstein's (1977) concept of classification.

Classification does not refer to what is classified but to the relationship between contents (Bernstein, 1977). The principle of classification determines the discourse that is transmitted and its relationship to other discourses within the curriculum. For instance, the relation between educational or midwifery knowledge and everyday knowledge, or between subjects. If the boundary between the contents is clear, Bernstein calls this strong classification (C+); if it is not clear, it is called weak classification (C−) (Bernstein, 1977).

Strong classification creates a powerful sense of membership and identity for students; they recognise the specialised knowledge as something sacred. Whereas, weak classification is less specialised knowledge and has a less specialised identity. This means that some forms of practice knowledge were more highly valued by students and mentors. Therefore, this chapter is important as tensions are noted between types of practice knowledge valued by the members of the Midwifery Committee of the NMC as well as some midwives and students in practice. Ramifications of the differences between weak and strong classifications will be discussed with examples given to explore these concepts and the types of knowledge.

This chapter incorporates the literature previously critiqued in Chapter 1 to show that the forms of practice knowledge (communication, clinical skills, and research) are valued by other health sector professions to varying degrees. They were also valued differently by individuals within this research. The implication of this is that what counts as valid practice knowledge changes and depends on the person, practice, and context.

3.1 Communication and interpersonal skills

The NMC (2006) review of pre-registration midwifery education questioned whether students were equipped to meet the needs of current and future women and their babies. The consultation asked for views on the knowledge and skills, including interpersonal skills and attitudes, necessary for students to qualify as midwives. Several key stakeholder organisations, which included the Department of Health and equivalents in Northern Ireland, Scotland, and Wales, and the Royal Colleges of Midwives and Nursing, made suggestions about requisite types of communication, and a comprehensive account of these skills was developed. Thus, five Essential Skills Clusters (ESC) were published (NMC, 2009). These include communication (NMC, 2009, p.31–37), initial consultation between the woman and midwife (p.39–40), normal labour and birth (p.42–48), initiation and continuation of breastfeeding (p.49–55), and medicinal product management (p.56–64). This is what students in my study and the UK were assessed against to qualify as midwives.

Despite being considered essential by the profession, collectively, the ESCs were criticised by the students for the repetition and amount of interpretation needed.

> I think a lot of mentors' struggle with them. I thought I'd just signed that one, so maybe I hadn't interpreted that one correctly as this one is so similar.
>
> (S8/T3/G2)

> Yeah, they do and they're forever asking, 'Well, what does that mean?' Or they're just so wordy and they sound similar.
>
> (S5/T1/G2)

Students and mentors alike recognised the potential of misinterpretation of the ESC. They were particularly critical of communication and breastfeeding skills as they were considered pervasive.

> Yeah, you know it's an effective communication: communicates effectively with all women and members of staff and blah, blah, blah.
>
> (S5/T1/G2)

> So, I think it's difficult sometimes as there's so many, you just look at the books [PADs] and page after page of tick box[es] basically.
>
> (S14/T2/G4S)

> All about breastfeeding, let's forget everything else.
>
> (S13/T2/G4S)

> Communication and breastfeeding.
>
> (S12/T1/G4S)

Each skill, worded in a slightly nuanced way, needs to be signed by the mentor. For instance, 'consistently shows ability to communicate safely and effectively with women' and 'communicates effectively and sensitively in a range of different settings' (NMC, 2009, p.31). With 45 separate statements on communication and 30 for breastfeeding, it is not surprising students thought this way.

The students did not dismiss communication skills as something irrelevant; they thought they already had these skills.

> We've also both had previous roles dealing with the public and people, and we've both had children, so a lot of the skills, I know about communication, listening, and those sorts of skills, that's life that's given those to us.
>
> (S44/T1/G10)

When students think they already have everyday knowledge, such as communication skills, the Bernsteinian (2000) notion of weak classification (C−) can be used to explore the status and implications for midwifery practice.

> I'll chat away to the woman fully aware the midwife will speak if you've said something wrong.
>
> (S21/T2/G5)

> I am never worried about going to speak to a woman or my communication, or being able to talk.
>
> (S5/T1/G2)

'Chat' and 'talk' signify non-pedagogic communication, and this implies the student is not aware in their communication with a woman whether they are putting her at ease, assessing her wellbeing, and utilising their midwifery knowledge to support the woman. The context of their communication, it appears, has not been recognised.

By contrast, when students say:

> Talk about it; it's like the depth of your knowldege, the depth of understanding, so you might be able to do a skill but being able to explain it to someone else or be able to talk about the research that underpins it that's where the layers of understanding are bought out.
>
> (S26/T1/G6)

The interpretation is that S26 understands the specific context of her communication. It is strongly classified from everyday knowledge (C+); she recognised the need to use a particular form of communication to support her explanation. Bernstein (2000) says the dominant modality of human communication is narrative, telling a story rather than analysis. When students 'just talk' to women, they are using a narrative form. When they explain and understand their communication, they are more likely to be using an analytical form. Students need to recognise the particular context of their communication to enable them to move from everyday communication skills (C–) to pedagogic communications (C+) with the woman or their mentor. They also need to be able to do this, as the NMC (2009) state, in a range of different settings. The latest NMC (2019) *Standards of Proficiency for Midwives*, that all students will need to demonstrate before entering the professional register, have communication skills embedded within every domain. Students explicitly need to communicate with women, their partners, families, and colleagues.

The assumption that students already have communication skills was reinforced by written feedback from many of the students' mentors. In the 19 three-year students' PADs reviewed, most mentors (n=17) commented on communication skills on the students' first placement. At the mid-point interviews, usually two or three weeks into the students' placement, seven students were noted to have good (S41/T3, S29/T2, Sk/T3, S39/T2, Sa/T2), effective (S1/T2), or excellent (S35/T2) communication skills in clinical practice. By the end of the first placement, ten students had positive comments about their communication skills. Two students had specific criticisms, 'increase awareness of own opinions and how these may conflict with those of clients' (Sn/T1) and, 'should be clearer in her communication by structuring discussions with women more logically and carefully' (S2/T1). Only two had no written feedback at all on their communication skills (S4/T1, Sb/T3), which could be interpreted to mean there were no issues.

A few students had areas of communication they needed to develop. These are noted to be in style, which was unrelated to the context and content, which was context-dependent. Five students needed to develop confidence in communicating, usually with women (Sj/T3, Sl/T3, S18/T3, S29/T2, S21/T3). Seven students had specific communication skills such as screening information, antenatal booking, and postnatal care advice that need developing, all feedback from the community setting (S35/T3, Sc/T3, S41/T3/ S29/T2, S2/T1, Sk/T2/ S39/T2). Skills noted to be necessary on the Central Delivery Suite (CDS) tended to be 'communicating with women in labour' (S1/T2, S35/T2) 'documentation and completion of paperwork' (S21/T2, Sa/T2), and 'terminology or vocabulary development' (Sa/T2, S35/T2).

When reviewing the seven 78-week students' PADs, similar comments from mentors were recorded. Three students had good communication skills documented within two weeks of starting midwifery practice, and one was noted to be effective with women and staff. By the end of their placement, one further student was considered 'good' (Sh/T1). Two others needed to develop confidence with their communication skills. As for three-year students, 'knowledge of screening tests' in community settings and 'communicating with women in labour' in the hospital were identified as needing development (Sv/T1, Su/T1). Therefore, despite the 78-week students being qualified nurses, similar areas for development and areas of strength were identified. It is this knowledge that is unique to midwifery and separate from nursing care; therefore, it is not surprising the feedback was similar for all students.

From the analysis of the PAD, it appears that a limited amount of written feedback is given to students on their communication skills. This reinforced the students' belief they were good communicators. However, as they progressed through their education, the expectation of whom they communicated with and a shift from verbal to written communication was observed.

> Liaises well with women and families and also other members of the multi-disciplinary team (MDT). Is providing woman-centred labour care and keeping contemporaneous labour records to a very high standard.
>
> (Mid-point interview: S29/T2 – first placement of the third year on CDS)

> An effective and appropriately confident practitioner. Works well and communicates within MDT.
>
> (Mid-point interview: Sj/T3 – second CDS placement third year)

> Excellent communication skills. Uses active listening to ascertain women's understanding of the situation. Communicates well with members of the MDT. Areas for development: To gain further experience liaising with the MDT, e.g. take part in case discussions, CTG meetings, handover etc. Take the lead in the handover of care and referral to obstetrician/paediatrician when appropriate. More experience of referring to MDT.
>
> (Mid-point interview: S19/T3 – first placement of the third year on CDS)

The 78-week students had similar feedback. However, the need to interact with the MDT and engage with the paperwork was documented sooner as their course is shorter. Due to their nursing qualification and experience, these students should already be more familiar with communication and documentation in clinical practice.

> To gain more confidence with the conversations with pregnant women, get more experience in the MDT, take more of a lead role in antenatal booking appointments, do birth plan.
>
> (Mid-point interview, written by a student in areas for development: Se/T3 – community placement, first six months)

One student during the group interview pointed out that mentors had different expectations about what and how documentation should be completed.

> Recently my documentation has been really criticised, which is fine I'm open to constructive criticism, and I have taken it on board, and definitely, I have improved since the criticism, but I don't think that mentors should turn

around and say that would be acceptable if you were working with so and so, but it's not acceptable if you're working with me.

(S1/T2/G1)

You're always going to get differences.

(S2/T1/G1)

The differences between midwives' practices, such as documentation style, can also be understood as strong classification. Therefore, from the students' perspective and from feedback in the PAD, what counted as valid communication skills changed depending on the environment and the people involved. This was summarised by two of the 78-week students.

> And the trouble ... is, while we know how to communicate depending on who you are communicating with [and] the environment, it will change and fluctuate on how you're feeling and all the rest of it. (S16/T1/G4S)
> And I'm sure you'd all agree that you communicate, depending on who you are working with some people you feel really, 'Oh God I can't say that', or do that and other people you get in it and you're there and you can just be yourself. (S15/T1/G4S)

The need to know the mentor's preferred style of communication affected how the student responded. This is an example of how the interaction between the student and mentor positively or negatively affects the amount and depth of communication between the individuals.

In the interviews, the mentors showed an awareness of the importance of both communication and interpersonal skills in judging students' practice:

> That's sort of how their demeanour is at work ... the language they use with women, whether it's professional ... a really good rapport with women ... what she's like when she comes out of the room.
>
> (M6/T2/C)

> Just sort of seeing how they are communicating with the women.
>
> (M8/T3/C)

It was one of the criteria mentors used to evaluate students' practice. Not divulging too much about themselves, chatting to women but not becoming a friend, and changing the information offered to accommodate the individual woman were also said. There were boundaries about the amount and nature of communication that students needed to recognise and adhere to. However, these were not always made explicit to the student and affected some students' ability to qualify. This will be discussed further in Chapter 6.

Some students expressed that they exhibited positive interpersonal skills.

It's something about the people skills that I feel I have that is so easily linked to midwifery and I always try to get that across, and I can't really explain it, but that's my thing, people skills.

(S39/T2/F9)

This too was reiterated by mentors in the written qualitative feedback in the PADs. Most of the comments were positive, such as good team working skills and well-liked by staff and women, or shows an aptitude, a pleasure to work with, and enthusiasm. Many of these comments were punctuated with exclamation marks or smiley faces, which I interpret to signify approval from the mentors of the students' persona. On almost every placement at the endpoint review, some positive aspect of the students' interpersonal skills were noted.

Has demonstrated a high level of midwifery skills and care. Has set clear goals and achieved them. Her ability to connect with women and provide a level of care is fantastic, midwifery skills that shine through. Has taken the lead role under supervision of admitting women and assessing their progress and caring for them to a high standard. Her teamwork is excellent from cleaning rooms with the support workers to assisting doctors confidently when seeing women; she should feel proud of her achievements. I am pleased with her progress. She shows a commitment to becoming a very good midwife, and I look forward to working with her in her second year. Well done!

(CDS first year S31/T3)

Her ability to learn rapidly has made her a pleasure to work with. She has developed rapidly towards being a confident and competent practitioner in the community setting. Her maturity, confidence and enthusiasm for midwifery has been evident throughout, and it has been a pleasure to mentor her. I have no doubt that she will continue to develop into an excellent midwife.

(Community first year S2/T1)

A pleasure to work with … Has sought opportunities to develop her skills … She has been able to work with minimal supervision, and this has enabled her to build her autonomous practice. Has worked hard at contemporaneous record-keeping while also caring and communicating with women. She communicates effectively as part of the MDT and is always keen to learn. She is a valued member of our team.

(CDS third year S39/T2)

One area for development identified regarding interpersonal skills was 'confidence and a belief in self'. This seemed to encourage students to be the midwife they wanted to be; to embody the role.

Trust your instincts; believe in yourself.

(CDS third year S4/T1)

Develop self into an autonomous individual midwife.

(Community third year T2/T1)

Myself and many of my colleagues hold the student in high regard; she is showing a real potential to becoming a brilliant midwife and a valued colleague of the future.

(CDS second year Sl/T3)

For the student to continue to work to this standard and more to enable her to practice as an autonomous practitioner.

(Community third year S19/T3)

She works well within the team and also has great empathy with the women. She is able to look after women with little support but knows when to ask for help if needed. She is working well to becoming a valued member of the team and good midwife.

(CDS 78-week final year Sg/T2)

Collectively, the positive comments about students' personas and the reinforcement to believe in themselves could be interpreted as foregrounding the individual rather than the commination and relational aspect of the role of the midwife. Comments about a perceived lack of confidence were also documented by mentors.

A lack of confidence can make her stand back; with greater experience her confidence will improve.

(Sf/T1)

Her confidence is growing, and she will ask for help or advice when appropriate. She still requires encouragement.

(Se/T3)

Overall, students who were proactive, able to work under indirect supervision, and needed less encouragement were valued in the practice environment. There was little feedback for most students on their communication and interpersonal skill, so the feelings expressed by the students that they already had these skills were reinforced.

Finally, some three-year students explained why they felt communication skills were not as important to them.

The first year is, as you know, treats women with respect, communicates well, and then by the time you get to the third year it still says the same thing and you kind of think, 'well'. (S9/T2/G3)

That's already been covered in the first two years. (S11/T1/G3)

If you're not doing that then you shouldn't be in the third year. It should be that you can competently catheterise, ARM [perform an artificial rupture of membranes]. (S9/T2/G3)

Yes, those sorts of practical things that there's nothing in the PAD about doing an ARM or catheterising is there? (S10/T3/G3)

When ... they're all the things that stress you out, you know you can talk to women and communicate, or you wouldn't be doing the job. (S9/T2/G3)

These vignettes illustrate that students were more concerned about practical skills than communication. They considered that students without the required communication skills should be failed and withdrawn from the programme. The students' opinion that there was no need to revisit basic communication skills each year seem valid from the documentation in the PAD. Only a few students had feedback about knowledge of screening choices or dietary information in their third year. However, their ability to communicate at a more sophisticated level each year was not fully appreciated. It was as if communication was a binary phenomenon, something you could or could not undertake, rather than something that developed with time and experience. The weak classification of this form of knowledge meant that not all students recognised the importance of the special context that they were in when communicating with women or mentors.

The professional literature related to this section will be considered later in this chapter because it encompasses all types of practice knowledge, not just communication and interpersonal skills.

3.2 Specific clinical skills

Students develop clinical skills by undertaking midwifery care supervised by their mentors. The skills discussed in the student interviews included:

1. Vaginal examinations
2. Venepuncture
3. Catheterisation
4. ARM or amniotomy
5. Continuous electronic fetal monitoring using cardiotocography (CTG)
6. Managing women's care with an augmented labour or epidural

There was a tension between what students wanted to practice and the vision from the regulatory body. Students wanted to practise the clinical skills they saw as necessary for their future practice as a qualified midwife. However, the NMC vision was for newly qualified registrants to be 'competent and confident in supporting women in normal childbirth' (NMC, 2009, p.17). As many of the clinical skills noted above are considered interventions in the normal birth process, they were debated during the NMC (2006, p.15) consultation process that reviewed the standards for pre-registration midwifery education. The respondents and key stakeholder organisations, described earlier, had divided opinions as to whether inducing or augmenting labour with an ARM (number 4 above), or syntocinon infusion (number 6), epidural for pain relief (number 6) and continuous monitoring of the fetal heart (CTG) (number 5) had a place within normal midwifery practice (NMC, 2006). Excluding these interventions was thought to compromise the ability of students to achieve their births, and they would be under-prepared for practice (NMC, 2006). Therefore, while not excluded there is only one mention of some of these skills within the standards: for entry onto the register, 'critically appraises and justifies the use of any intervention, such as artificial rupture of membranes, continuous electronic fetal monitoring, urinary catheterisation, in order to facilitate a spontaneous vaginal birth' (NMC, 2009, p.49). (This has position has changed in the NMC (2019) standards and will be addressed later in this chapter.)

For this reason, perhaps, the students were dismissive of the standards as they did not prepare them for 'real practice'.

> It should be more about the practicalities of the job than conforms to the NMC standards; you know … I don't think the PAD document … reflects what you do in practice. What we're scared about is 'Oh my God, I've got to look after a woman with an epidural or synto [syntocinon infusion]'.
>
> (S9/T2/G3)

Specific midwifery skills were also noted in an Australian study of 19 student midwives (Licqurish and Seibold, 2013). The focus on normal births meant students felt less confident with specific skills including vaginal examinations, urinary catheterisation, documentation, medication administration, and dealing with emergencies (Licqurish and Seibold, 2013). Catching a baby was not considered to involve a lot of skill, especially if a hands-off approach was used and some of the skills such as vaginal examinations, students felt, should be recorded (Licqurish and Seibold, 2013).

The students were interviewed before and after their final placement, and their competency assessment documents were used to support the discussion (Licqurish and Seibold, 2013). Five students were also observed in practice; however, no discussion of this data is provided in the publication. While the reasons for difficulty in gaining the number of births differ between Australia and the UK, the pressure some students felt was similar. In Australia, three-year direct-entry students spent 30–42 weeks in clinical practice, while the students in my study had 67 weeks. The difficulty in gaining normal births was attributed to competition with other students, rising levels of interventions, and some control of birth by obstetricians in private hospitals (Licqurish and Seibold, 2013). These difficulties were not expressed in my research; students were accepting of one another's needs.

> The priority was the third years that hadn't had the births … which I know we're going to have that when we come into the third year.
>
> (S35/T1/G8)

However, the NMC (2009) focus on normality reduced opportunities for clinical skill development as this newly qualified midwife explains three months after qualifying:

I had all my deliveries quite early on, and I'd seen a lot of normal, which is why I'd had my deliveries early on. I really felt I needed to expose myself to more abnormality … I really felt that we needed that, and I have been proven right. And [there's] still so much I haven't done because I did see so much normal. There's so many different abnormalities aren't there? You can't possibly have seen everything … There's still things I have never had, no shoulder dystocia yet you know, I've had little PPH's [post-partum haemorrhages] but nothing dramatic, I've just seen very normal. So, there's a load I feel I need to learn.

(S45/T1/G10)

S45 switched pronouns, most of the time she used the singular, *I*, talking about her experiences, but she also used the plural '*we needed that*', to signify students generally articulated the necessity of more exposure to clinical skills and high-risk midwifery cases. The former student used *just*, stressing she has only seen normal midwifery. She believed her lack of complex and high-risk experiences had not prepared her for midwifery practice.

Mentors also seemed to value students who could undertake specific clinical skills.

I said, 'Oh we need to do a CTG', she'd got it all ready, and she'd been out and got someone to sign it. 'You're just brilliant. How's the partogram looking?' 'Yes, it's all up to date'. 'That's brilliant'. It's a pleasure to have someone working with you like that; you are more working like a team.

(M11/T1/H)

There were reasons why mentors wanted students to be exposed to the more specialised clinical skills.

So, IV [intravenous] drugs for example, now I know they [students] can't give IV drugs, but you can get involved in making up syntocinon or antibiotics because as a student, my biggest fear was that someone was going to shout that I need 40 units of synto[cinon] quick and was me thinking 'Ohh', whereas if they get routinely into the habit of making up the synto … when they qualify, it is going to be easier.

(M7/T2/H)

I am talking about a third-year now, if, for example, you ask a student to prepare everything, we need for … a syntocinon infusion and they are going and doing and preparing everything. You know they know what you need … if you've got someone who doesn't know and they will take one thing and a few minutes later will go and bring you another one, so that it looks like they are not really sure, if you would prepare everything at the same time you know this person knows and has got it.

(M15/T2/H)

Not only was it considered necessary in an emergency for students to be able to help, and it aided their transition to qualified practice, but it was used to stratify students into those familiar with clinical skill preparation from students unfamiliar with the processes, even though it was not a requirement of the regulatory body (NMC, 2009). Here a lack of congruency between the pre-registration midwifery curriculum informed by the regulatory body's vision, students' clinical experience and mentor expectations is noted. This causes a tension in what counts as valid practice knowledge between agents.

In the PAD, mentors often wrote about clinical skills, but these tended not to be the skills the students considered important. Some of the skills, like communication skills, were context-specific. In almost every first-year PAD, mentors commented about basic midwifery skills.

> Competent at basic observations T, BP, P [Temperature, Blood Pressure and Pulse], palpation of the size of the uterus, presentation, location of heartbeat, and using Pinards [stethoscope].
> (Mid-point interview: S31/T3 first community placement first year).

> Basic clinical skills developing well. Areas to work on: BP, urinalysis, palpations, auscultation of FH [fetal heart].
> (Mid-point interview: S4/T1 first community
> placement first year)

> Developing antenatal skills such as palpation, BP, P, FH auscultation. Areas to work on: To continue to develop skills such as BP, P and palpation, begin to take part in NBST [new-born screening test].
> (Mid-point interview: S41/T3 first community
> placement first year)

The skills the students wanted to develop were not documented in their PADs until the third year, except for vaginal examinations (VEs); however, these still needed development in the final year.

> Continued to develop practical skills such as VE's and ARM. Actively involved in medicines management. Areas to work on: Needs to develop confidence in her skills.
> (Mid-point interview: Sl/T3 MLBU penultimate
> placement third year)

> Drugs, FSE [fetal scalp electrode], ARM, cord gases, paperwork, perineal repair.
> (Student identified areas to work on: Sm/T3 first
> placement of third-year CDS)

Student is performing all her skills to a high standard and gaining confidence all the time. Areas to work on: I have no concerns regarding her practice, as yet to perform ARM or FSE and these are skills she would like to practise if the opportunity arises. Has attended two perineal repair workshops and is now ready to perform uncomplicated suturing with direct supervision.

(Mid-point interview: S29/T2 third year CDS placement)

Sanderling University midwifery students were not the only UK students to feel they lacked specific clinical skills. Newly qualified midwives in Wales were noted to feel unprepared to undertake important midwifery skills, including venepuncture and amniotomy (Darra et al., 2016). Darra et al. (2016) identified 16 specific skills not documented by the standards (NMC, 2009). Concerns that newly qualified midwives were expected to, and felt the need to, undertake certain skills they had not developed and practised sufficiently, lead the four universities in Wales to develop a passport that students completed alongside the NMC competencies (Darra et al., 2016).

In my study, the 78-week students did not mention technical competences in the interviews, possibly because they had already developed many of these skills in their nursing careers. Only one 78-week student was noted to need experience in conducting an amniotomy in their PAD (Sg/T2). However, the three-year students emphasised and valued technical skill acquisition. They were more critical of the 'promoting normality agenda'. Their perception was that the current standards did not prepare them for the reality of the next stage of becoming a fully independent midwife.

Using Bernstein's theories (2000), clinical skills can be interpreted as strongly classified (C+). The skills were recognised by the students as special midwifery knowledge. This type of practice knowledge was highly regarded and sought after, especially by the three-year students. McIntosh et al. (2013, p.1182) called these 'hard' skills; students noted them to be 'concrete and observable' and capable of being taught and practised in a clinical setting or skills laboratory (McIntosh et al., 2013, p.1182). Soft skills, such as communication were valued less (McIntosh et al., 2013); perhaps because they were weakly classified. McIntosh et al. (2013) undertook in-depth focus groups with 120 final year midwifery students from six UK universities to explore their experiences of learning how to become a midwife. Like my research, the authors note tensions between the regulatory body's vision, practice learning environments, and university philosophies. Four themes were identified from the students, two of which are relevant here. Students did not think they were taught enough for their future role, and they were keen to learn practical or clinical skills, especially hard skills (McIntosh et al., 2013). Concrete skills were considered essential, while psychological issues were regarded as optional extras. This can be understood as the difference between strong and weak classification of the skills.

The mentors, however, with the lack of written feedback in the PADs, could be interpreted as having a relaxed attitude towards skill acquisition. Students were given the opportunity to practice the basics, blood pressure, pulse, temperature, and abdominal palpation, early in their education. However, the skills the students most wanted (numbers 3–6 at the beginning of this section) were often only available to students in the final year. The impending transition from student to peer appeared to have an impact on the emphasis of gaining clinical skills. The interpretation of this is that students are progressively socialised into the midwifery profession, and the integration process enables access to the sacred, special knowledge. However, full access only seems available towards the end of their education.

The latest NMC (2019) *Standards of Proficiency for Midwives* include most of the skills students are concerned about. These include; vaginal examination with the woman's consent, venepuncture, cannulation and blood sampling, amniotomy, the application of fetal scalp electrode, auscultation of the fetal heart, using Pinard stethoscope and cardiotocograph (CTG), and providing midwifery care for the women and new-born infant before, during, and after medical interventions, including epidural analgesia, instrumental births, and caesarean section (NMC, 2019). While the skills are explicitly stated, access to these may still depend on where students are in their education in terms of placement area and year of practice and the midwife they are working with.

3.3 The use of research to inform practice

Another content of the curriculum is to prepare students to use evidence to inform practice (NMC, 2009, p.5). I believe research is one aspect of the curriculum that should transcend theory and practice boundaries, as midwives need these skills to provide evidence-based care. As all the students were taking undergraduate studies, and some of the mentors were undertaking degree and masters' study, I was expecting more comments about the application of theory and research evidence to support practice knowledge. However, there was an assumption from the interviewees that students had more time than qualified staff to read and understand research. Research seemed slightly peripheral from midwives' daily practice and thus not necessarily seen as valid midwifery practice knowledge, despite being a professional requirement, as these quotes show:

> And quite often they [mentors] say to us students because we have time to read and we do read the latest journals and research that we go in and they might be talking about something like when the whooping cough vaccine came out, we kind of knew more about it than the midwives on the ward did because they hadn't been informed about it as much as we had.
>
> (S20/T2/G5)

> There have been cases where … a midwife has been talking to somebody, and maybe, I wouldn't say it in front of the woman, but maybe I'd say

afterwards, well we recently covered this and this has slightly changed now or something, or I was reading something and they [mentors] are usually very receptive to that.

(S19/T3/G5)

She [the mentor] was trying to teach me sterile technique, and I was like sorry we don't do that anymore and just sort of said we've been taught to do it this way ... but you have to be very careful how you do it.

(S14/T2/G4S)

We [mentors] give them an opportunity to talk about areas of research, and I think, and I'll always say to a student right at the very beginning of working with them, if you think I'm not doing something or there's been some new evidence out, please let me know because the students are far more up to date with new guidelines and evidence than what a lot of midwives are.

(M5/T2/C)

I think they [students] can help us sometimes because they talk about research, what they are doing. Quite a lot has been talked about the third stage, and I know they've been doing that at college, so it's really interesting to hear. So, I think it keeps us [mentors] up to date, they develop us.

(M6/T2/H)

This student I've had recently I would always tell her to put a jaundiced baby in sunlight, and she said to me there's this research that's come out to say that's not actually effective anymore. So, I say to her I would love to read it.

(M9/T3/C)

These findings, from mentor and student interviews, suggest that students have more time and are better informed about research than midwives are, and some can share this knowledge. However, S14 had a cautious approach when discussing best practice with her mentor.

In the interviews, the midwives' attitudes towards research knowledge seemed to be reliant on the students keeping them informed, rather than the mentors informing the students about the latest evidence-based care. The group mentor interview did not spontaneously talk about research, so I asked:

And what about when the students come to you and say have you read this new research? Do you think you can then have a conversation with them, and they can [interrupted]? (SCM).
[Names M10], stop pulling faces? [Laughter] (M11).
Do they not say that to you? (SCM).
No, no one has said that to me (M11/T1/H).
No, they don't, I'd quite like them to really (M12/T1/C).

They never say that, I've never had a student say that to me, never (M11/T1/H).

I'm just trying to think now. No, they just go along, don't they? They're training, but I don't feel like I am ever challenged by a student (M10/T1/H).

OK (SCM).

Do you? (M10/T1/H).

No, not really. I expected it more, 'why did you do it like that?' (M12/T1/C).

But when they do, they're confrontational, or are they? Do you know what I mean? They can't win; they can't win (M10/T1/H).

I was hoping that they'd be coming to me telling me new things that I didn't know about, but not so far (M12/T1/H).

The dialogue shows that not all students and mentors have discussions about research evidence. In the PADs, other mentors documented how they had either discussed or been informed by students; these comments were usually from the community mentor.

I have learnt from her knowledge which she shares gently.

(Sn/T1 community mentor)

Openly shares her knowledge with the other team members. Reflects on her own practice and seeks to better her knowledge.

(Sa/T2 community mentor)

Shares knowledge and questions midwifery practice. Is aware of different styles and ways of practising.

(S39/T2 community mentor)

Some mentors discussed evidence, especially the NICE (National Institute for Health and Care Excellence) guidance. Few mentors named any specific guidance, rather they used NICE as a generic term. NICE produces guidance on many aspects of nursing and midwifery practice which informs care options and are evidence-based. One mentor said midwifery practice changed frequently:

And I think lately it's been so many new research about all sorts of different topics that you sort of sometimes you feel that six months ago we were doing this and that and now it's changing because there has been some research and that. So yeah, I think it's learning all of the time. But I think it is just updating more than like a proper when you need to sit and properly look through your book and do some work. I think it is more like updating your knowledge.

(M15/T2/H)

She explained how she personally maintained her research knowledge:

Well I do the guidelines and the policies we've got in the hospital [names a few policies] so when your updating the guidelines you are looking through what is out there, you are looking through NICE, and you're looking through RCOG [Royal College of Obstetricians and Gynaecologists] Guidelines, you need to obviously read them to be able to compare what we've got in our policy and what's out there.

(M15/T2/H)

This mentor had a master's degree, which may be why she was chosen to be part of the guidelines group in the first place, and this work in turn kept her up to date. She had also completed her midwifery education in an EU country and commented upon how lecturers worked with students in clinical practice and questioned their research knowledge more than mentors in the UK. Therefore, her research was integral to her identity as well as role. However, M9/T3/C explained her distance from the guidelines and perhaps research knowledge in practice:

If there was any guideline that you could use, maybe use them and obviously if, we haven't got access to them because often in the community we don't always have a computer present obviously make sure they [the student] know where to find them. Perhaps give them that to go away and do.

(M9/T3/C)

Here, the difficulty of accessing the guidelines in the community is a barrier to facilitating up-to-date research knowledge. Instead of considering the evidence together, perhaps due to the lack of computer access, the mentor sends the student away to read and learn from guidelines independently. This activity physically separates the student and the evidence from the work midwives engage in and could symbolically reduce the relevance or value of research to inform practice.

Other midwifery research and expert opinion supports the idea that midwifery care is based on traditional midwifery practice and clinical experience rather than evidence-based practice (Hunter, 2013; Armstrong, 2010; Bluff and Holloway, 2008). In the qualitative study of 20 students and 17 qualified midwives, Bluff and Holloway (2008) noted two types of role models for students: prescriptive and flexible. The prescriptive midwives tended to use traditional knowledge rather than evidence to inform practice. As students generally emulated the practice of their role models, and the prescriptive midwives tended to be more experienced and have status and position, students often practiced as they instructed. The flexible midwives enabled the students to better understand the rationale for care and develop their own style of practice (Bluff and Holloway, 2008). The effect role models have on students can affect the development of the student, and attention needs to be paid to learning appropriate behaviours that also impact upon the care women receive (Bluff and Holloway, 2008). A limitation of this research is that it was undertaken over several years. However, as the next chapter will show these types of midwives prevail, and some midwives do not seem to use evidence to inform practice as obviously as others.

When discussing evidence-based care with student midwives in Wales, the consensus was that not all care practices are grounded in evidence (Hunter, 2013). Drawing on her extensive experience as a midwife and researcher, Hunter (2013) considered two barriers to using evidence-based practice. First, questioning traditional practices is not encouraged, and second there is a 'black box' to implementing research into practice. Hunter's (2013) black box had four components. First, the quality and accessibility of the research was seen as a potential barrier, but organisations such as NICE and the Cochrane Collaboration, now critique and summarise key research and make recommendations for practice. Therefore, research is now more accessible. Second, some organisations and professions were not ready for change. Next, some issues are more important than others, so these changes occur. Lastly, using evidence to support her discussion, Hunter (2013) says practitioners' personal experiences may limit the application of research into practice but reducing the gap between researchers and knowledge users, she believed, would improve the application of evidence-based care.

Two of Hunter's (2013) barriers were seen in my study: organisational and personal experience. Organisationally, the 'Trust's way' (M7/T2/H) was noted to be a barrier to implementing evidence-based care. However, not all midwives at this Trust supported this. Thus, midwives personal experience affected their engagement with the evidence. M15 noted there were many changes to practice, and she was close to the research evidence with her role on the guideline development group. However, M9, in the community, expressed limited access to evidence which may have distanced her further from the research.

Regarding Hunter's (2013) first challenge, evidence from the PAD presented earlier showed that some students could question midwives' practice. Perhaps these are the so-called 'flexible midwives' (Bluff and Holloway, 2008), or the student has established a good working relationship or has a particular style that enables them to do so. More discussion on the relationship between students and mentors is offered in the next chapter. Positive examples of the integration of evidence to inform practice were noted in some students' PAD.

> Works with evidence-based practice and questions why and when we work as we do.
>
> (Sv/T1)

> Questions policy, procedures, and practice appropriately to ensure evidence-based.
>
> (S1/T2)

Thus, it seems some students have access to research knowledge and can also discuss this with their mentor.

The overwhelming impression in my study was that students were more up to date than their mentors. This concurs with a study of 125 student midwives from five universities in the UK (Armstrong, 2010). Ninety-two per cent of students agreed that the evidence taught in university did not correspond to their experiences in clinical practice, and 76% said their mentors suggested ways of practising that were different to the evidence (Armstrong, 2010). Students thought that the clinical environment was too busy to implement evidence-based practice (39%), that policies and guidelines were not evidence-based (52%), and they did not have the authority to change practice (78%). Students did not challenge their mentor's practice for fear of jeopardising their clinical assessments (Armstrong, 2010). None of the students in my study expressed the relationship between their practice grade and challenging a mentor; however, caution was noted earlier in how students did this, perhaps because they understood this had the potential to change how mentors evaluated them as a person.

It would seem that students and mentors differ with respect to how explicitly evidence is used to inform practice. The Bernsteinian (2000) interpretation is that a minority of midwives have an integral relationship with the evidence base as part of their role, thus a weak classification (C–). However, the majority see utilising evidence to inform practice as more peripheral or something separate to their role, so counterintuitively the classification is strong (C+). From a student perspective, knowing and understanding the evidence is part of their university studies and should be central to their student identity; hence, weak classification. As students' progress through their course, they tend to adopt the views and identify with the qualified staff so may start to distance themselves from the evidence base (C+). As a profession that considers itself evidence-based, this has ramifications for midwives' and students' identity. The latest NMC (2019) *Standards of Proficiency for Midwives* has many key themes running through the domains; the first of these is evidence-based care and the importance of staying up to date with current knowledge. However, as midwifery has been an all graduate profession for over a decade and this form of practice knowledge is still strongly classified as separate from many midwives' roles, it remains to be seen whether these standards alter this. That said, the rapid change that has occurred in midwifery practice as a result of the Covid-19 pandemic and growing body of evidence that has informed these changes, including joint publications from the Royal College of Midwives (RCM) and Royal College of Obstetricians and Gynaecologists (RCOG) may have a long term positive effect on the midwifery profession with regard to utilising evidence-based care.

3.4 The literature: valid practice knowledge

Much of the literature from healthcare professional education critiqued in Chapter 1 described the types of knowledge necessary for practice. Table 3.1 shows the types of practice knowledge assessed by the different health professions. If the profession assesses the form of knowledge, one can deduce that type of practice knowledge is valued.

The first point to note, from Table 3.1, is the marked similarity between the health professions regarding valid practice knowledge. The types of knowledge

Table 3.1 Types of practice knowledge assessed

Type	Professions	References
Communication and interpersonal skills	Nursing, midwifery, medicine, physiotherapy	Oermann et al., 2009; Smith, 2007; Clouder and Toms, 2008; Briscoe et al., 2006; Murphy et al., 2014; Imanipour and Jalili, 2016; Eggleton et al., 2016; Fisher et al., 2017; Hanley and Higgins, 2005; Meldrum et al., 2008.
Cognitive/ evaluative abilities (Clinical knowledge or evidence-based practice)	Nursing, physiotherapy, medicine, pharmacy, midwifery	Oermann et al., 2009; Clouder and Toms, 2008; Briscoe et al., 2006; Manning et al., 2016; Imanipour and Jalili, 2016; Lurie and Mooney, 2010; Murphy et al., 2014; Eggleton et al., 2016; Fisher et al., 2017; Scammell et al., 2007; Meldrum et al., 2008.
Psychomotor and technical skills	Nursing, midwifery, medicine	Oermann et al., 2009; Smith, 2007; Briscoe et al., 2006; Scammell et al., 2007; Imanipour and Jalili, 2016; Eggleton et al., 2016; Meldrum et al., 2008.
Values, attitude and professional behaviours	Nursing, physiotherapy, medicine, pharmacy	Oermann et al., 2009; Clouder and Toms, 2008; Briscoe et al., 2006; Manning et al., 2016; Murphy et al., 2014; Susmarini and Hayati, 2011; Imanipour and Jalili, 2016; Eggleton et al., 2016; Scammell et al., 2007; Meldrum et al., 2008.
Safe to practice, safety	Midwifery, nursing, physiotherapy	Smith, 2007; Clouder and Toms, 2008; Murphy et al., 2014; Amicucci, 2012; Docherty and Dieckmann, 2015; Scammell et al., 2007.
Self-management	physiotherapy	Clouder and Toms, 2008; Meldrum et al., 2008.
Skills (but not determined which)	Pharmacy, nursing, physiotherapy, midwifery	Manning et al., 2016; Susmarini and Hayati, 2011; Lurie and Mooney, 2010; Clouder and Toms, 2008; Fisher et al., 2017; Scammell et al., 2007.
Punctuality	physiotherapy	Clouder and Toms, 2008.

can be broadly categorised into Bloom et al.'s (1956) three learning domains: affective, cognitive, and psychomotor. Categorisation of types of knowledge can be restrictive, so caution must be stated here. It is also acknowledged that the content of the communication and specific skills used in each profession will change; however, most professional health programmes seem to require students to demonstrate similar generic competencies.

Problems were noted in the studies with assessing practice knowledge (Briscoe et al., 2006; Smith, 2007; Clouder and Toms, 2008). Six types of practice knowledge were identified and explored to demonstrate their usefulness for assessing medical students (Briscoe et al., 2006). The survey of medical school directors in the US (n=85, response rate 66%) described discrepancies between types of practice knowledge and their usefulness. In descending order, attitude, professional behaviour, interpersonal skills, communication skills, clinical skills, and clinical knowledge were judged to be 'very useful' by respondents (34.6–24.7%, respectively). The emphasis was on skills in the affective domain. The main way the affective domain was assessed in the large-scale US nursing survey was through faculty observation of students with patients (67%) or with others (54%) (Oermann et al., 2009). However, the frequency of observation, by whom, reliability, and validity were all questioned in Chapter 1. Therefore, many healthcare professions utilised a range of methods of assessment.

When asked what the perfect clinical assessment tool in medical education would entail, clinical skills, professional behaviour, and clinical knowledge were cited most frequently; however, there was little agreement between respondents (Briscoe et al., 2006). The hypothetical question awarded higher significance to clinical knowledge than the usefulness grade of 'moderately useful' (Briscoe et al., 2006). This could be an example of the participants offering socially desirable responses. Clinical knowledge should, one could argue, feature more significantly in the assessment of students, but it seems even in medicine the affective domain and the style of the person counts for more. A similar number of medical directors said clinical knowledge was either 'minimally useful' or 'very useful' (24.7%, respectively) in the clinical assessment. This survey illustrates there is no consensus about the usefulness or importance of assessing distinct types of knowledge, and it varies according to individuals.

3.5 Midwifery practice knowledge

In Smith's (2007) qualitative study of 12 midwifery mentors, when asked what the students' practice grades were based on, communication skills and psychomotor skills were cited most often. How well the student related to others and dexterity were important. However, when asked about research knowledge, mentors were impressed with students' ability to access it, with no discussion of its evaluation or application to midwifery practice. Thus, some students were awarded grades for motivation rather than a critical appraisal of the evidence. One participant said, 'we're not a very good research-based resource, we're experience-based' (Smith, 2007, p.115). Another participant, however, actively sought discussions with students about research, but most of the grade was from the clinical performance (Smith, 2007). The differing mentor identities with respect to research align with my study.

In the wider midwifery literature, all forms of practice knowledge, discussed above, communication and interpersonal skills, specific competences, and using evidence to inform practice are identified specifically in relation to what it means to be a good midwife (Carolan, 2013, 2011; Nicholls et al., 2011; Byrom and Downe, 2010; Nicholls and Webb, 2006).

First-year midwifery students in Australia, like the students in my work, expressed the personal qualities they possessed that were essential for midwifery practice (Carolan, 2011). The 32 direct-entry students, questioned after five weeks on the course, considered interpersonal skills were necessary to build relationships with women (Carolan, 2011). When asked again two years later in a separate study, the remaining 30 third-year students identified being a skilled practitioner, interpersonal skills, and passion underpinning their perceptions of a good midwife (Carolan, 2013). Clinical competence, based on research supported by continuing professional development was as important as the affective qualities of caring, compassion, and enthusiasm for midwifery. Thus, evidence for midwifery practice was combined with interpersonal skills.

Carolan (2013) observed the third-year students seldom discussed the importance of communication skills. Her interpretation of this omission was that communication skills may be so integral to being a good midwife that the students may not have thought they warranted mentioning (Carolan, 2013). Her interpretation differs from my research. I hypothesise students do not seem to value communication skills because they are weakly classified and that they already possess them, and this is reinforced by comments in the PAD. However, specific types of communication did need improving, including documentation, referring to the multidisciplinary team, and planning care.

A limitation of both studies (Carolan, 2011, 2013) is the method of data collection. Although some quantitative demographics are stated, and vignettes from qualitative statements are used, it is not clear whether the students were interviewed as one group, several groups, or individually. Carolan (2011, 2013) states the data was collected the week after a group information session, so one might assume a group interview was undertaken. However, with 32 and 30 students, respectively, this might not be the best approach to enable all participants the opportunity to participate. The implications for practice are clear though. Initially, students displayed a limited view of the role of the midwife (Carolan, 2011). By the third year, students' views better aligned with qualified midwives, but there was a lack of emphasis on the importance of communication skills (Carolan, 2013).

At the point of registration, Butler et al. (2008) identified three necessities for student midwives: being safe, having the right attitude, and effective communication skills. The emphasis is on the affective domain. In their study of 39 qualifying midwives and assessors and 20 experienced midwives across six universities, less emphasis was placed on clinical skills as some midwives understood the need to develop those once qualified, such as vaginal examinations (Butler et al., 2008). While the data was collected over a decade ago, before the current changes to pre-registration midwifery education were introduced (NMC, 2009), the work still has some relevance today. The mentors in my research documented in the PADs the student's ability to ask for help thereby being safe, and their positive attitude and communication skills. However, there is perhaps a greater pressure for new registrants to have specific clinical skills as noted by the Darra et al. (2016) and the participants in my study.

When the qualities of a good midwife are considered in more detail, the need for effective communication skills is more apparent than technical skills (Nicholls and Webb, 2006). In order to develop midwifery curricula, an integrative review of 33 research papers on definitions of a good midwife were reviewed by Nicholls and Webb (2006). Eight concepts were identified from the literature, including the attributes of a midwife, what a midwife does and research. The midwife's personal qualities and good communication skills made the biggest contribution from the literature, which used a wide range of different approaches and methods (Nicholls and Webb, 2006). Due to the lack of research on 'what makes a good midwife' their follow-up study used a Delphi questionnaire (Nicholls et al., 2011). They questioned 226 postnatal women, midwives, and midwifery educators who collectively deemed effective communication skills, lifelong learning, and individualised care as the most notable features of a good midwife (Nicholls et al., 2011).

The research differentiated between the three participant groups, and there was consistency between their perspectives (Nicholls et al., 2011). However, the recruitment of women to the study was via an email from the National Childbirth Trust, so this may have limited participation to those with internet access, and the group were self-selecting which means their views may not represent those of other women. A further limitation is that the second round of the Delphi had a poor response rate (38%) (Nicholls et al., 2011). There was no discussion on the communication finding in Nicholls et al.'s (2011) paper, so its value on what or how communication is needed is limited. Nonetheless, the implication is that tailoring care to individuals relies on good communication to enable women to make choices informed from the evidence (Nicholls et al., 2011). Thus, once qualified, the importance of clinical skills seems to reduce, as the registrant presumably becomes accomplished with these.

In a phenomenological study of ten midwives' views of the characteristics of a good midwife (Byrom and Downe, 2010), personal qualities were valued as much as skill competence. Skilled competence included clinical skills, but it was not stated which specific midwifery skills, rather the generic terms clinical or practical skills were used. The personal qualities encompassed communicating in diverse ways with different women to form a relationship. The midwives were selected from a random sample of junior and more senior staff, so a wide range of perspectives were heard (Byrom and Downe, 2010). However, the study was not wholly focused on being a good midwife as being a good leader was also considered, there seemed to be some overlap between these roles though, and both needed practical competence and interpersonal traits (Byrom and Downe, 2010). As the findings support the two previous studies there seems to be consensus on what a good midwife is.

When the views of women on what makes a good midwife were collected, immense importance was placed on the relationship between the two (Borrelli, 2014). Borrelli (2014) selected and critiqued six studies, four with a qualitative approach and two surveys with a range of participants including couples, nulliparous, and multiparous women (n=19–825 participants) from four countries (England, Australia, Sweden, and USA). Having choice and feeling in control was necessary, and for that women needed appropriate information. This study shows women's perspectives do not wholly align with the midwives' perception. Rather the need for good supportive relationships aligned with the first-year students' perspective presented earlier (Carolan, 2011).

From the literature, and my research, what counts as valid midwifery practice knowledge seems to *depend*. It depends on who is asked, and it differs between service users, students, and midwives, it is also different between areas such as community or delivery suite. It also seems to depend on the stage of training the student is at (Carolan, 2011, p.2013). The reasons why some practice knowledge is valued more than others can be understood using Bernstein's concept of classification.

3.6 Classification and its application to midwifery practice

The concept of classification can refer to the degree of insulation between agents, practices, and contexts (Bernstein, 1977). Classification is used here to explore the nature of knowledge in the midwifery curriculum. Strong classification is used for agents, subjects, and contexts that have clear boundaries. Whereas, weak classification refers to less clear-cut boundaries.

Regarding the agents, the boundary between the women, students, and midwives can be explained by strong and weak classification. Initially, the first-year students' views of a good midwife align more with those of women than with those of the profession (Carolan, 2011). As students progressed, they see themselves as more like midwives (Carolan, 2013). Carolan (2013) noted one student spoke of herself as a midwife, rather than a student. Her interpretation of this was that the student was developing her midwifery identity with the blurring of the line between being a third-year student and qualified midwife. Bernstein would call this weak classification. Initially, there is a weak classification between the woman and student and strong classification between the student and midwife. At the end of their education, the classification between woman and student is strong as students are more like midwives, and the classification between third-year students and midwives is weak. The classification strength, therefore, evolves with professional socialisation of the student, with implications for teaching, learning, and assessment which will be discussed in the next chapters.

Differences were also presented regarding the types of communication practices first and final year students were expected to demonstrate. In the first-year students were expected to build a rapport with women and then offer information, such as screening choices. In the third year, more emphasis was placed on documentation and interactions with the multidisciplinary team as legitimate communication practices. As students' progress in their studies, the insulation between them and the midwives reduces, this is weak classification, as the student takes on more of the midwifery roles such as documentation.

The problem with communication skills was that students did not always recognise this form of midwifery practice knowledge as specialised knowledge. Many students expressed a minor difference between communicating in everyday life and communicating with women; the skills were similar, thus it was a weak classification. However, midwifery communications with women are a specific context that is strongly classified from having coffee with friends. If a student does not recognise the specialised context they are in, they may demonstrate inappropriate talk and conduct.

The classificatory principle provides the key to the distinguishing feature of the context, and so orientates the speaker to what is expected, and what is legitimate in that context (Bernstein, 2000, p.17). Without explicit feedback from mentors about the forms of midwifery communication, there was a tendency for students to assume their communication skills were developing as expected; for many, this was the case. However, they may have developed further with more feedback to enable all students to recognise the specific context and form of communication required with women, other midwives and the interprofessional team.

It was rare for students later in their course, especially third years, to have specific areas of communication for development documented in their PAD, such as screening information. The interpretation is that they should already be able to demonstrate this form of communication early in their first year. However, confidence to liaise with the MDT and contemporaneous documentation was observed more often. If, at the end of the students' education, the classification is strong between them and the midwife, they are not yet like the midwife, it signified that the student was not performing as they should be.

Another practice discussed was undertaking clinical skills. It was clear to students when they were undertaking specific tasks, such as venepuncture and vaginal examination. They recognised that they were undertaking midwifery specific work. The students saw the acquisition of these skills as essential for their future careers. There was strong classification between these skills and everyday life and between other forms of midwifery practice. The interpretation of this is that there is a hierarchy regarding different practices. For the students, access to the clinical skills was most important, especially at the end of their course. Within this hierarchy there were skills first years could undertake; blood pressure and abdominal palpation, whereas more specialised skills, such as induction of labour, were not introduced until the third year.

Some students thought they had everyday communication knowledge; therefore, they did not necessarily value communication skills as much as clinical skills. While the two skills should come together, underpinned by evidence, often the evidence was not seen as midwives work. Thus, using evidence to inform practice can be interpreted as strongly classified as students' work rather than practice knowledge necessary for all midwives.

Following Bernstein in his reference to Durkheim, the difference between communication skills and specific clinical skills can be understood in terms of the sacred and profane. The clinical skills were highly prized because they were specialised midwifery practices initially inaccessible to the student. Access to these skills came later in the students' course. The focus on normality in the students' education was distinct from what the students were expected to do as newly qualified midwives; thus, this agenda was criticised by the students because it did not prepare them for the reality of practice. In Bernsteinian terms, this would be strong classification. The boundary between being a student and focussing on normality is clearly different from that of a qualified midwife. The new NMC (2019) *Standards of Proficiency for Midwives* have moved away from students focussing on normality. They explicitly include communication and specific midwifery skills, with a greater focus on research and caring for women and babies with additional needs. This should better prepare students for the realities of qualified practice; however, it is too soon to know how these will be received and recontextualised by midwives in the clinical environment and affect the next generation of midwives.

Some evidence was presented that individual midwives had diverse ways of working and of conceiving what was acceptable and what was not; thus, the boundary between these agents can be strongly classified. Students had to understand the midwife's practices to recognise her preferences and produce a legitimate performance. This will be explored further in the following chapter. Similarly, the boundary between the contexts, such as the type of care offered in the delivery suite was different from the care in the community. The expectations of students and skills necessary in these areas were context-specific. This is a strong classification and this will also be discussed further.

This chapter has discussed three types of knowledge needed for midwifery practice: interpersonal and communication skills, clinical skills, and evidence to inform practice. Students and mentors seemed to give more value to clinical skills and facilitated the achievement of these more overtly than the importance of communication skills. There was a reticence about discussing research with students, and this may give students the impression this is not 'midwives' work. Midwives do adhere to the NICE guidelines which are evidence-based, but it seemed this was embodied knowledge 'we do it like this' rather than a critical stance on the research.

Students interpersonal skills, putting women at ease, team working, and enthusiasm were ways they demonstrated embodiment into their professional role; however, some students saw this as everyday rather than midwifery specific knowledge. Students' interpersonal skills were positively commented upon in the PADs, with explicit punctuation which foregrounded their personas, rather than the way they used communication skills or evidence.

Clear divisions were noted between the regulatory body's vision of a newly qualified registrant and the actual knowledge needed for practice, which led to some areas of knowledge being highly valued and others overlooked.

Bibliography

Amicucci, B., (2012). What nurse faculty have to say about clinical grading. *Teaching and Learning in Nursing*, 7(2), pp. 51–55.

Armstrong, N., (2010). Clinical mentors' influence on student midwives practice. *British Journal of Midwifery*, 18(2), pp. 114–123.

Bernstein, B., (1977). *Class, Codes and Control Volume III*. 2nd ed. London: Routledge.

Bernstein, B., (2000). *Pedagogy, Symbolic Control and Identity Theory, Research, Critique*. 2nd ed. Maryland: Rowan and Littlefield Publishers, Inc

Bloom, B. S., Engelhart, M. D., Furst, E. J., Hill, W. H., Krathwohl, D. R. (1956) Taxonomy of educational objectives; the classification of educational goals, Handbook 1 : Cognitive Domain, New York, David McKay Company.

Bluff, R. & Holloway, I., (2008). The efficacy of midwifery role models. *Midwifery*, 24, pp. 301–9.

Borrelli, S. E., (2014). What is a good midwife? Insights from the literature. *Midwifery*, 30(1), pp. 3–10.

Briscoe, G. W., Carlson, D. L, Arcand, L. A, Levine, R. E. & Cohen, M. J., (2006). Clinical grading in psychiatric clerkships. *Academic Psychiatry*, 30(2), pp. 104–109.

Butler, M., Fraser, D. & Murphy, R., (2008). What are the essential competencies required of a midwife at the point of registration?. *Midwifery*, 24, pp. 260–269.

Byrom, S. & Downe, S., (2010). 'She sort of shines': Midwives' accounts of 'good' midwifery and 'good' leadership. *Midwifery*, 26(1), pp. 126–137.

Carolan, M., (2011). The good midwife: Commencing students' views. *Midwifery*, 27(4), pp. 503–507.

Carolan, M., (2013). 'A good midwife stands out': 3rd year midwifery students' views. *Midwifery*, 29(2), pp. 115–121.

Clouder, L. & Toms, J., (2008). Impact of oral assessment on physiotherapy students' learning in practice. *Physiotherapy Theory and Practice*, 24(1), pp. 29–42.

Darra, S., Wyn-Davies, J., Edgerton, L., Morse, N. & Thomas, G., (2016). Working to implement a pre-qualifying skills passport in Wales. *British Journal of Midwifery*, 24(7), pp. 478–483.

Docherty, A. and Dieckmann, N., (2015). Is there evidence of failing to fail in our schools of nursing? *Nursing Education Perspectives*, 36(4), pp. 226–231.

Eggleton, K., Goodyear-Smith, F., Paton, L., Fallon, K., Wong, C., Lack, L., Kennelly, J., Fishman, T. and Moyes, S., (2016). Reliability of Mini-CEX Assessment of Medical Students in General Practice Clinical Attachments. *Family Medicine*, 48(8), p. 624.

Fisher, M., Bower, H., Chenery-Morris, S., Jackson, J. and Way, S., (2017a). A Scoping Study To Explore The Application And Impact Of Grading Practice In Pre-Registration Midwifery Programmes Across The United Kingdom. *Nurse Education in Practice*, 24, pp. 99–105.

Hunter, B., (2013). Implementing research evidence into practice: Some reflections on the challenges. *Evidence Based Midwifery*, 11(3), pp. 76–80.

Imanipour, M. and Jalili, M., (2016). Development of a comprehensive clinical performance assessment system for nursing students: A programmatic approach. *Japan Journal of Nursing Science*, 13(1), pp. 46–54.

Licqurish, S. & Seibold, C., (2013). Chasing the numbers: Australian Bachelor of Midwifery students' experiences of achieving midwifery practice requirements for practice. *Midwifery*, 29(6), pp. 661–667.

Lurie, S. J. and Mooney, C. J., (2010). Relationship between clinical assessment and examination scores in determining clerkship grade. *Medical Education*, 44(2), pp. 177–183.

Manning, D. H., Ference, K. A., Welch, A. C. and Holt-Macey, M., (2016). Development and implementation of pass/fail grading system for advanced pharmacy practice experiences. *Americal Journal of Pharmaceutical Education*, 8(1), pp. 59–68.

McIntosh, T., Fraser, D., Stephen, N. & Avis, M., (2013). Final year students perceptions of learning to be a midwife in six British universities. *Nurse Education Today*, 33, pp. 1179–1183.

Murphy, S., Dalton, M. & Dawes, D., (2014). Assessing physical therapy students' performance during clinical practice. *Physiotherapy Canada*, 66(2), pp. 169–176.

Nicholls, L., Skirton, H. & Webb, C., (2011). Establishing perceptions of a good midwife: A delphi study. *British Journal of Midwifery*, 19, pp. 230–236.

Nicholls, L. & Webb, C., (2006). What makes a good midwife? An integrative review of methodologically-diverse research. *Journal of Advanced Nursing*, 56(4), pp. 414–429.

NMC, (2006). NMC Consultation, *'Review of Pre-Registration Midwifery Education'*, *Decisions*. London: Nursing and Midwifery Council.

NMC, (2009). *Standards for Pre-Registration Midwifery Education*. London: Nursing and Midwifery Council.

NMC, (2019). *Standards of Proficiency for Midwives*. London: Nursing and Midwifery Council.

Oermann, M., Yarborough, S. S., Saewert, K. J., Ard, N. & Charasika, M., (2009). Clinical evaluation and grading practices in schools of nursing; national survey findings part 2. *Nursing Education Perspectives*, 30(6), pp. 352–357.

Scammell, J., Halliwell, D. and Partlow, C., (2007). *Assessment of practice in pre-registration undergraduate nursing programmes: An evaluation of a tool to grade student performance in practice*, Bournemouth: Bournemouth University.

Smith, J., (2007). Assessing and grading students' clinical practice: Midwives lived experience. *Evidence Based Midwifery*, 5(4), pp. 112–119.

Susmarini, D. and Hayati, Y. S., (2011). Grade inflation in clinical stage. *American Journal of Health Sciences*, 2(1), p. 21.

4 Learning and teaching in clinical practice

This chapter looks specifically at teaching and learning, the valid transmission and acquisition of knowledge, in clinical practice. The key theme identified in the empirical data was the centrality of an effective relationship between the student and mentor. Students placed great emphasis on acquiring practice knowledge and explained how a relationship with the mentor enabled or prevented access to this knowledge. The hierarchy between the student and mentor was a feature of the relationship. Some students understood how they could alter the hierarchy with the mentor and enacted this to enable greater access to learning opportunities. The approach of mentors to facilitate learning in the clinical environment lead to positive or negative labelling by students: good or dreaded. Similarly, mentors discussed types of students in relation to how easy or hard they were to teach.

The acquisition of knowledge depended on recognition of the learning activity. However, distinct types or categories of students held contrasting views with respect to recognising the learning in clinical practice, due to weak or strong classification. Two methods of learning, role modelling and acquisition of clinical skills, are explored in detail to show how teaching in clinical practice can be implicit and/or explicit for different students.

Differences were also articulated regarding the learning activities between contexts: within the hospital or community settings. Busy clinical environments, especially within the hospital setting, were a barrier to knowledge transfer from midwives to students as the work rather than the learning was prioritised. The students perceived overstretched hospital midwives observed less of the students' practice. In the community, relaxed mentoring relationships and time in physical proximity with the midwife were common experiences. These differences affected student knowledge acquisition.

Examples will be given from the empirical data: from student and mentor interviews and quotations from student PADs. Themes are supported by UK literature on teaching and learning in clinical practice, especially in relation to midwifery education.

The work of Bernstein (1990, 2000) has been drawn upon to explore the social relations between mentors and student midwives and how knowledge is transmitted and acquired in clinical practice. For knowledge to be demonstrated, students must recognise and then realise a specific legitimate performance within that context. Recognition comes from the classificatory principle, introduced in the previous chapter but expanded upon here to demonstrate how it can impair acquisition of practice knowledge. Realisation of the appropriate performance is dependent upon framing.

Framing refers to the principle regulating the communicative practices between acquirers and transmitters (Bernstein, 1990); in my study, specifically between students and their mentors. Where framing is strong the mentor regulates the features of the communicative context. When framing is weak, the student has more control. The features of the communicative context include the selection, sequence and pace of learning and its evaluation or criteria. The strength of each feature is independent, so some features may be strongly framed and others weakly. Variations in the framing principle, whether they are strong or weak, regulate variations in the realisation rules (Bernstein, 1990). The realisation rule is the capacity to demonstrate the appropriate practice, within a specific context.

4.1 Establishing effective student–mentor relationships

Establishing effective working relationships was the first of the mentors' responsibilities outlined by the regulatory body in Supporting Learning and Assessment in Practice (NMC, 2008). This has been superseded by the NMC (2018) *Standards for Student Supervision and Assessment*. While the explicit requirement to establish relationships no longer exists, midwives do need to serve as role models for safe and effective practice and support students to learn (NMC, 2018).

In the relationship between the student and mentor, the acquirer must learn how to be a student, and the transmitter should learn how to be a mentor. Mentors, due to the asymmetric relationship with students, are in a hierarchical position (Bernstein, 2000); however, they can reduce the hierarchy to support student integration in the workplace.

From the student data, mentor behaviours were described that helped students feel a sense of belonging or alternatively, contributed to their outsider status.

> They know you are there and they'll say, 'Hello' but they don't actually involve you with what's going on.
>
> (S40/T2/G9)

> They say, 'Oh, I've got a student today!' I say I have got a name … We're just called 'a student'. I don't like being called 'a student' … You know if you're in the staff room, you're not involved, they are just talking among themselves, and you feel a bit alienated, don't you? A good mentor will just join you in the conversation.
>
> (S42/T3/G9)

On the ward, you've got the board, and it's got all the different areas and say it will have who is working in each bit and she'll [the mentor] put your name up there. And you're like, 'Oh God, my name is on the board'.

(S39/T2/G9)

[My mentor] puts my name first on the board with the lady, so your name first. You're looking after her; the mentor is helping you.

(S41/T2/ G9)

Students describe small actions that help them feel included or excluded in the clinical environment. Mentors who knew students' names and used them to show who was caring for each woman, and who initiated conversations in the spaces outside the clinical care environment helped students feel part of the team. This seemed to reduce the hierarchy between mentors and students. The last quote symbolically demonstrates the learner as in control, rather than the mentor. (It also demonstrates the power of language used in practice versus that of the university. In university, students are taught to use the term woman; however, in practice the use of the word lady seems to prevail).

Most students articulated the need to get to know a mentor for a day or two to establish a relationship.

I think … you need a couple of shifts just to build up a relationship with the mentor, you need that.

(S36/T2/G8)

I feel quite fortunate because I've had a bit more stability, so I've been able to build up a bit more relationship with my mentors.

(S27/T1/G6)

I think when you're in practice, and you're with a mentor for 40 or whatever per cent you are with your mentor, it is personal because you build up a mentor-student relationship and they look at you in practice every day, and it's every aspect. It's your communication, what you are actually doing what you are doing for the baby, for or the mum, your written documentation.

(S48/T2/G11S)

Note how S36 stressed the necessity of building a relationship by using 'need' at the beginning and end of the sentence. It is central to accessing practice knowledge. S48 recognised that her manner was scrutinised in the way she talks, practices, and documents care. Recognising this meant the student had understood or read the context, and this orientated her to what was expected or legitimate in that context. The difference between S42's account (above) and S48's can be explained by strong and weak framing. S42 was called 'a student'; she was referred to by her position. Her identity and its lower status relative to the registrant was foregrounded when her name was not used. This is a feature of strong framing. By contrast, S48 says her relationship with her mentor is 'personal'; the student is an individual rather than a position. This is symbolic of weak framing.

While most of the students were acutely aware of the importance of their relationship with the mentor, few of the mentors spontaneously voiced their opinion or measures to actively establish this. Instead, mentors were more concerned about students building relationships with the women (M7/T2/H; M14/T2/H).

However, some midwives reflected upon their experiences as students.

> It is quite a nice thing to have that relaxed relationship with a student because I think they're, that if they have any problems, they will perhaps open up a little more, and I can remember as a student like the example I give of the pots in the wrong place, that sort of thing, it's not nice to have that relationship.
>
> (M9/T3/C)

M9 purposefully created a relaxed relationship with students. Recognising her learning was negatively affected by the experience she espoused a more positive mentoring style. Other mentors too, explained how they were mentored, and this affected their current mentoring style. Most mentors expressed a preference for a reduced hierarchy between them and the student.

> We are friends … I see them as colleagues really.
>
> (M8/T3/C)

Conversely, some students were concerned about other students' relaxed relationship with a mentor.

> I do worry some people are really friendly.
>
> (S5/T1/G2)

> Like they're bringing their friend along rather than their mentor.
>
> (S8/T3/G2)

> Yeah, because of course you've got to have a good relationship, but where do you stop at a good relationship and you know socialising with your mentor? Not that I do.
>
> (S5/T1/G2)

> I know it sounds awful as they [mentors] like us all but if they like you as a person and want to go out and have a drink with you and want to be your friend they're 100% more likely to give you fantastic grades.
>
> (S20/T2/G5)

Others who had this weak hierarchy valued it.

> The two mentors whom I have mainly worked with are a similar age to me, and one of them gave her my email address, and she has been emailing me stuff about things to do with practice, and so it's almost been like we're sort of friends more than professional sort of relations (S32/T1/G7).
>
> Do you worry about that? (SCM).
>
> Not really … I had her sort of more for emotional support if you see what I mean? That's why she did it, and I was glad that she did (S32/T1/G7).

In a traditional teacher–student relationship, the teacher is usually older. However, in midwifery, student and mentor ages can be similar, and this may facilitate a closer relationship. The reason why some students were concerned about others' relaxed relationships with mentors is that they thought this conveyed some advantage. However, as students progressed through their education, the hierarchy between them and the mentor often decreased as the classification between them weakened, and they moved from outsider to insider status. With less difference between the role of a midwife and student about to qualify (C–), the framing strength of the hierarchy between the student and mentor also tended to weaken (F–).

4.1.1 *Ineffective working relationships*

Mentor characteristics were described; however, some constituted ineffective relationships and students did not want to work with these midwives.

> You've got good mentors and the dreaded ones … If you end up with someone who isn't supportive of you, you know, that you don't get on with or you clash with for whatever reason, then that is six weeks out of your life that you are going to dread going to work every single day.
>
> (S14/T2/G4S)

> I had a mentor, on one of the placements, and she was just so negative, so negative … the way you said, 'Good morning' you could be completely wrong … You don't learn because you are so nervous, and it's like your mind is closed.
>
> (S49/T2/G11S)

> My mentor, nine times out of ten, will be [deliver a baby] hands-on and this other mentor was hands-off, and she was like, 'Why are you doing that?' In front of the woman too, it's like now the woman thinks that I don't know what I'm doing.
>
> (S34/T1/G8)

> So, I found it really difficult and ended up having the grumpy mentor, but I mean she's just very sour-faced, and everybody knows that she is grumpy. It's

to the point where I mean she's always trying to get rid of you; she doesn't want you working with you (S30/T1/G7).

How does she get rid of you? (SCM)

Sends you to the pharmacy, sends you everywhere that's not near her. She'll have her break and then she'll come back, and she won't have her break with you. So, it's almost like another block of time not with you. She'll do the drug round, and I'll be, 'Oh I'll come along' and, 'Oh no, it's only a few meds [medicines]'. She'll just get rid of you. Other students that have worked with her have all said the same. I tried to not have her (S30/T1/G7).

There are multiple examples of labels for ineffective midwifery mentors in the literature such as controlling (Hughes and Fraser, 2011), over-protective (Fraser et al., 2013), unwelcoming (Kroll et al., 2009), unhelpful (Longworth, 2013), as well as bad mentors (Holland et al., 2010). Collectively these studies researched (n=493) midwifery students and newly qualified midwives (n=35) across the UK, London, Wales, East Midlands. The aims, scope and size of the research differed; however, the centrality of the role of the mentor to accessing practice knowledge and behaviours that enabled or inhibited this were prevalent in all studies. Two of the studies are introduced here, the others relate to points later in the chapter.

The largest, multi-site, multi-method, case study, sponsored by the NMC, evaluated the contribution midwife teachers, working in universities, brought to outcomes for mothers and babies (Fraser et al., 2013). As the research was commissioned by the profession's regulatory body, one could question whether its findings would be more susceptible to bias than non-commissioned research. However, a range of researchers and collaborators were on the project team, and the study included views from a range of stakeholders, including students (n=165) on both three-year and shortened programmes, and newly qualified midwives (n=35) whose views align to my work and others. The inference is, therefore, that the potential bias of this study is minimal. Students gave verbatim examples of when their mentor 'takes over, so you don't learn' (Fraser et al., 2013, p.50) and 'don't allow you to do it' (p.54) when discussing negative mentor behaviours. Students particularly disliked working with midwives who disparaged them in front of women (Fraser et al., 2013; Hughes and Fraser, 2011). This is consistent with S34's comment above.

Hughes and Fraser (2011) studied student midwives (n=58) views on the role of the mentor in practice, and survey of the qualities they needed was conducted in one university in the East Midlands. A strength of their research is the longitudinal aspect. Data was collected from two successive cohorts of students on three or four occasions during their three-year course. Their experiences and learning needs changed over time; however, there was general agreement on the qualities of a good mentor. Students wanted to be able to ask their mentor questions, and for their questions to be explained, to be encouraged by their mentor, and give the student time to learn new skills (Hughes and Fraser, 2011). These characteristics led to the term 'guiding hands'. Mentors who were less helpful were perceived to be more controlling of the student. Using similar phrases as the students in the Fraser et al. (2013) research, these mentors did not enable students to 'move forward' or progress (Hughes and Fraser, 2011).

While relationships are bidirectional, it was often incumbent upon the student to improve the relationship with their mentor, which enabled greater access to learning.

> One particular midwife that I was working with, she completely ignored me really. I thought right let's see if we can do this, so she had to take a bed down to the bay, and I said, 'I'll help you'. I went running down and held it. I thought I am going to find something that we've got in common, it just happened to be Slimming World, and I was like OK we've found this in common, and we hit it off fine, ever since then we've been absolutely fine, but I thought I've got to crack her because otherwise it's going to be awful. I do find it a bit of a challenge sometimes.
>
> (S42/T3/G9)

This student felt the mentor had ignored her. She used the collective term: we. She recognised that both she and the mentor needed to be invested in her education for it to work. She knew she had a better chance of her educational needs being met if she could get the mentor to see her as 'someone like her' by trying to find something in common. She altered the framing strength from strong (positional) to weaker (personal). The common activity is irrelevant; it is getting the mentor to see the student as a person so they can then work together. The term 'crack' as in under psychological pressure is quite an extreme word; however, it seemed to work. Since that interaction, the student says the relationship with the mentor was fine, but the effort was on the student to establish this. This is reiterated by other students.

> Sometimes simple things like a bed needs changing and jump to go do it first, they [mentors] love it when you change a bed. It's like on the birthing unit I was working with a different midwife, and you just be overly helpful and just go and do everything and then it might annoy them, but at the same time it might make them realise you are there and that works.
>
> (S39/T2/G9)

S39 knew that recognising the work and completing it before the mentor could was one way to be noticed, although she noted there was a risk to this. Both students (S39 and S42) could alter their access to learning opportunities because they understood how to become visible to the mentor.

In any pedagogic relationship, the hierarchy can be explicit or implicit. If they are explicit, the power relations are clear, and the student is in a position of subordination and mentor superordination. Many mentors and students preferred a relaxed hierarchy, and this seemed conducive to accessing and acquiring practice knowledge. However, there were mentors who were more authoritarian; some of their behaviours seemed to suppress practice learning. Some students could alter the framing strength from strong to weak and positional to personal, which enabled greater access to learning opportunities. However, not all students were able to, and for S30, presented above, this affected her ability to learn midwifery. Her case is presented in Chapter 6.

4.2 Recognising the teaching and learning in clinical practice

When asked how they were taught, three categories of student responses were noted:

1. Those who were nurses first,
2. Those with previous healthcare experience, and
3. Those with no prior healthcare experience.

The 78-week students recognised transmission and acquisition of knowledge in clinical practice.

> You observe and then they'll [the mentors] observe you perform that task, and then you'll perform that task and then if you're confident you will continue doing that or if you felt you needed more time you need to be able to say actually, can we go through that again and again or however many times you need to do it, and then they watch you excel throughout your placement in that specific task.
>
> (S48/T2/G11S)

> So, when you are watching them, them being the mentors, are you just watching them or is something else happening that is part of a teaching process? (SCM).
>
> We're asking questions (S47/T1/G11S).
>
> And they're explaining why (S48/T2/G11S).

Whereas, the students who had healthcare experience felt midwifery practice knowledge needed more explaining.

> I let them know I was a support worker before so teaching was like, 'Oh you should know this, you've worked in care before so you should know this', I feel I wasn't given that much info compared to others who were fresh into it …
>
> (S31/T3/G7)

> The first day they asked what you did you do before this? The truth is well I was a care assistant, and they'd go, 'Oh excellent, so you can do this and do this', before having any explanation as to why or if anything is different. They'd just say can you do obs [observations] on this person and this person and they need to be done every 15 minutes for the next two hours, you'd be like … OK then.
>
> (S29/T2/G7)

I was a support worker beforehand, but on my first day on the ward, I was really nervous, and I think that was very portrayed in me. They [mentors] were really good actually and took me back to basics. I wasn't a support worker in the hospital I was in someone's home, so it is a lot different, but yeah, they were very good very basic and nice and slow, and if I got it, it was move onto the next thing.

(S30/T1/G7)

The experiences of students with no earlier knowledge were most varied.

How are you taught in clinical practice? (SCM).

By just mucking in and getting on with it (S41/T2/G9).

Are you taught? (SCM).

Yeah but I think it is experience taught as well. I won't say that it's taught this is literally what we are going to do. Maybe in the beginning and you hadn't seen anything they [the mentors] can talk you through it but not actually talk it through while the procedure is going on but discussing it afterwards or before. I think a lot of it is just experience taught (S40/T2/G9).

I've never had that. I've never had somebody talk me through anything.

(S41/T2/G9)

I was always asked to be the first time, regardless.

(S39/T2/G9)

See for me I wasn't a support worker, so going in the first thing they taught me as I was on the ward first was to do the obs [observations] and things like that, and then they said to me, 'Right you can have that bay for today', and obviously, I was supervised but I went around and felt really independent very quickly, and it felt like they had a lot of trust in me very quickly, so that was quite a positive thing for me.

(S28/T3/G7)

There was general agreement above from the 78-week students that acquiring practice knowledge was dependent upon observation of their mentor's practice, practising themselves, and questioning their mentor to understand or improve their performance. They recognised the learning process. As many of these students had been mentors previously, they may have been better prepared to answer such a question. Some of the students considered their earlier healthcare experience detrimental to learning midwifery. These students felt like they were quickly part of the workforce without more explanation. This left these students wishing they had not said anything about their earlier experience (S31); wanting more explanation but reluctantly accepted tasks (S29), and grateful her need for further support was enabled (S30). Some 78-week students also wished they had concealed their prior identity, 'You're a nurse first … that's great I can give you all these jobs to do' (S14/T2/G4S) because it potentially limited their learning.

Some of the activities, such as undertaking clinical observations, are shared by healthcare assistants and nursing registrants. However, the role and responsibility of a midwife is fundamentally different from that of a care assistant, and the differences should have been articulated to the students, as S29 alluded to. The doxa of the profession was already partly shared by both types of students. They understood the 'natural order' of healthcare environments and work. Therefore, mentors may have assumed that these categories of students already had the requisite knowledge, and this limited their exposure to further learning opportunities as they took part in the workload.

This is partially corroborated in Kroll et al.'s (2009) study, undertaken as concerns were raised about the learning environment on the postnatal ward between 2005 and 2007. Opportunities for learning were available on the ward, but students' workload often prevented them from accessing these (Kroll et al., 2009). Midwives thought shortened course students were quicker to learn than three-year students and therefore needed less support on the postnatal wards (Kroll et al., 2009). Although 71 student midwives were invited to participate, and 49 agreed, there is no differentiation of the year of study or type of course they were on (Kroll et al., 2009). Neither were the differences in the responses from senior midwives, nurses, or midwives articulated (Kroll et al., 2009). This is a limitation, but it could be due to the short word count of the journal.

In my study, students with healthcare experience, 78-week students, and S28 with no previous experience felt an expectation to contribute to the workload, without due attention paid to their learning. While S28, positively valued undertaking the observations and felt independent, as for her this was new knowledge and therefore a valid learning opportunity. For the other students, it was not new and therefore, not a learning experience.

The students with no previous healthcare experience had mixed encounters with practice learning. S41, especially, believed she had not been taught, and her mentor had not explained what was needed of her. She seemed to rely on her own common sense to decide what was right. S40, at first, had some explanation; however, she reported halfway through her course that there was limited discussion between her and her mentor. Whereas S39 explicitly asked the mentor to elaborate. These findings have some relevance to Longworth's (2013) mixed-methods study of student experiences of skill acquisition in the skills laboratory and clinical practice. While not wholly related to practice learning the comparison is offered to show how teaching is more visible in the university setting than in practice.

Questionnaires to 36 students from all three years were administered prior to an in-depth interview with six purposely selected students; half of these were in their third year (Longworth, 2013). The quantitative data confirmed university lecturers consistently taught the background to each skill (100%) and demonstrated it adequately (94%) compared to fewer explanations from mentors about the procedure (79%) (Longworth, 2013). The majority of students

(73%) said they had to work hard to get access to practice skills in the clinical area (Longworth, 2013). Despite this, many students thought learning in clinical practice was more relevant (Longworth, 2013). Positive qualitative comments were noted on recognising and developing skills depended upon mentor support and the relationship; however, unhelpful mentoring styles were barriers to students' learning (Longworth, 2013, p.835).

If students are unable to recognise the specific context they are in and learn from it, they are unlikely to demonstrate a suitable performance. It is the relationship with the mentor that guides students towards practice appropriate for the role. An example of an inappropriate first-year interaction shows how this student, according to the mentor, had clearly not understood the context she was in.

> 'What position is it in'? 'It's doing the splits'. In front of the woman, you know, and reading Heat magazine … and being too friendly.
>
> (M10/T2/H)

The student, it seems, had not recognised her words, activities, and behaviour were inappropriate. Without explicit feedback to that effect, she would be unable to show a more professional persona next time. Interestingly, the student left the course after six months, citing wrong career choice, perhaps the feedback on her professional behaviour disrupted her identity or orientation to midwifery.

4.2.1 Differences between the 78-week and 3-year students

Aiming to explore differences between students on the two courses, I asked the group of three mentors what they saw. M11 exemplified the paradox of mentoring the 78-week students.

> Because they've just got, they know how to be with people in the setting, and they've obviously got the basic skills as well, and you don't have to explain every little thing to them. I mean there were a couple that are mature students that have been very high up in their [nursing] area, but they've come to us and said don't worry about that, 'This is new for us'. At first, when I got a student that was a nurse, a post-grad they're going to think I am stupid because I don't know about nursing things, but they don't. They are really ᐧ good.
>
> (M11/T1/H)

> I am always pleased to have a previous nurse because it's an extra pair of hands as well isn't it, and they've already gone a long way.
>
> (M12/T1/C)

M11 reasoned that the 78-week students already possessed the necessary communication, interpersonal, and clinical skills. The assumption made here was that these students did not need to be taught these aspects of practice. However, they do need to be taught specific midwifery knowledge. M11 admitted she was worried by her lack of nursing knowledge as a direct entry midwife; the implication is she was worried about her own performance. The 78-week students seem to understand this and mitigated their mentor's apprehension when they explained that they were new to the midwifery arena. Students illustrated in the interviews the types of phrases they would use to enable them access to new learning opportunities:

> I'm halfway through, but midwife is completely different to everything I've been doing.
>
> (S16/T1/G4S)

> I am a novice midwifery student.
>
> (S12/T2/G4S)

M12 acknowledged students with experience reduced the mentor's workload as care could be shared.

While not said by any interviewee, there is the possibility that mentors may also feel inhibited and therefore worry about their teaching ability with experienced healthcare workers or students who have previously been doulas or breastfeeding support workers. This may also limit how much knowledge is transferred to these students.

4.2.2 Role modelling as a teaching strategy

When mentors were asked how they taught midwifery, most named 'role modelling' as their primary teaching strategy. Some had narrow definitions, such as students could 'model themselves on what midwives are saying to the women' (M12/T1/H). Others had a more holistic view:

> I want to always provide good role modelling whether that's with the woman or as a professional midwife. I would say the same about being part of village life or with my children, that for me good role modelling is a big part of my life, so I would certainly do that with students.
>
> (M5/T2/C)

The following student extract illustrates effective mentor role modelling.

> I had a mentor who was really quite a quiet person. She was the sort of midwife I'd want if I was having a baby and I learnt a lot from watching her, in terms of the way that she was with the woman and the way she approached things and the way she communicated and spoke to that woman, but she didn't really teach me. I just learnt those basic skills from her and then the odd sort of bit she'd go through like let's check the placenta together then

again, she wouldn't teach it, but she'd say, 'Well we look for this, and we look for this and this'.

(S28/T3/G7)

While this student clearly admired the midwife and learnt from her, she did not recognise the mentor's practice as a teaching strategy. Thus, the interpretation the student had is the midwife did not teach her.

Finnerty and Collington (2013) explored role modelling as one teaching strategy in their research using a discourse analysis of 14 second- and third-year student midwives' audio diary entries. They postulated, using cognitive apprenticeship as a theoretical underpinning, that role modelling is the first learning activity whereby the expert performs the skill and the student learns. Other elements of the model are coaching, scaffolding, fading, articulation, reflection, and exploration (Finnerty and Collington, 2013); although not all are illustrated in the publication. Scaffolding is where the mentor supplies individual feedback and guidance. Fading is where mentor support is gradually removed, placing the emphasis on the learner.

Presenting 8 of the 14 student audio diary excerpts, three which involved role modelling, Finnerty and Collington (2013) note all three students recognised some of the learning. However, for one student, they suggested there was more to the interaction than the student noticed. This can be understood using Bernstein's weak classification and can also be interpreted from S28's account; she understood she learnt interpersonal qualities from her mentor, but did not recognise when individual guidance was used to teach her how to examine a placenta.

Data for Finnerty and Collington's (2013) research was collected during a national study, published in 2003, so one could question the relevance of the research to contemporary practice; however, their findings resonate with students' learning experiences today. Especially the omission of fading by mentors (Finnerty and Collington, 2013). This is a feature of strong framing and seems to hinder student development, especially later in their educational journey. As not all students perceive these strategies as helping their learning and mentors may not move from one strategy to another, more learning conversations may be needed to enable all students to develop their potential.

One of the mentors in my study explained how she role modelled a practical skill.

> If it's a practical skill, I'd teach them. I'd go through it without a woman present, you know and make sure they know for example, if we're doing venepuncture or something go through what equipment you would need. Go through if there were any guidelines that you would use … And then obviously, observation of getting them to observe you to do it and then obviously let them do it under direct supervision and sometimes with a bit of help from you as well I think and then obviously, just then slowly step back … based on what the student is showing.

(M9/T3/C)

Her terminology on direct and indirect supervision and slowly stepping back is reassuring in that this implied she knew her role in the facilitation of learning (NMC, 2008, p.20) to 'use the student's stage of learning to select appropriate learning opportunities to meet individual needs'. This commitment is still present in the NMC (2018) Standards: learning experiences are tailored to the student's stage of learning, proficiencies, and programme outcomes.

The first stage of role modelling the skill is explicit, then M9 coaches and scaffolds the student by supplying guidance without the woman present and an opportunity to practise the skills. Depending on the student's competence, the mentor can adopt the fading technique leaving the learner in control. The frequency of the word 'obviously' implies there is no other way to or it is clear or visible what she has done, yet, as already said, while it might be clear to this mentor, it is not always for the student.

Students and some mentors recognised that copying their mentors' practice was sometimes necessary; this is different from role modelling: this is imitation.

> Because sometimes you need to know the things that the midwife prefers to do and you have to remember who is doing it that way, and you have to do it in that way with that particular person and in a different way with another person.
>
> (S47/T1/G11S)

> I think a student becomes very adept at transforming her practice to whom she is working with.
>
> (M5/T2/C)

Learning the mentor's preferences was most necessary when the mentor was explicit about how the student should practice. Knowing which criteria were important to the mentor meant the student could demonstrate a legitimate performance within that pedagogic relationship. These mentors are more likely to the 'prescriptive' mentors described by Bluff and Holloway (2008).

Bluff and Holloway (2008) said emulating the behaviour of prescriptive midwives was easy for students because those midwives made their expectations clear. Their approach would be interpreted by Bernstein (2000) as strong framing, 'this is how you do it' (Bluff and Holloway, 2008, p. 305). However, the term emulates means trying to be as good as or matching the practice of, and the students did not always value these midwives' practices. The prescriptive midwives tended not to use evidence-based practice; therefore, my interpretation is that the students could copy their behaviour but would not know the rationale underpinning it. The status, position, and authority of some of these midwives was a barrier to student learning.

Role modelling flexible midwives who offered a more woman-centred approach was harder for students (Bluff and Holloway, 2008). Their style could be interpreted as weak framing where a number of options are available for the student to decide from. The powerful effect of role models in midwifery are noted by Bluff and Holloway (2008), and attention is needed to prevent students from learning inappropriate behaviours.

4.2.3 Role modelling inappropriate professional behaviour

In my study, inappropriate role modelling was expressed more vehemently than positive behaviours.

> The biggest problem there is people bitch behind one another's backs, and actually, when you are walking down the ward at night, you don't want to hear one of the senior midwives bad-mouthing one of the other midwives, and I don't know I have always bought my children up that you should treat people how you want to be treated.
>
> (S44/T1/G10)

This student had just qualified so was less guarded when talking about the behaviour of midwives than some of the current students. She seemed more upset that it was a senior midwife whom she expected more of. She did not want to hear her talk about another member of staff in a negative way.

Unprofessional midwifery behaviours were reiterated by mentors when asked.

> Do you feel that the qualified midwives are good role models for professionalism? (SCM).
>
> No, not always I think some are. I think the difficulty is that as a qualified midwife you know … that there's some forums where you are safe to say certain things … that people have to … let off stress you know in a certain environment. You also know that the qualified midwife is then going to look after a patient and be totally professional. I think the trouble is that the students are at a level where they don't necessarily recognise the difference. So, I think in that way we are not always good role models we need to be more mindful of the fact that students are there and what we say in front of students. But equally I think they [students] need to know the realities of working. I think we are good role models in patient care when we are actually doing it, but I think in the non-clinical area maybe, we are not so much (M1/T3/H).

In another Trust, the same opinion was offered.

> Do you think all midwives act as good role models for professional behaviour? (SCM).
>
> Not all of them.
>
> (M12/T1/C)

> It's difficult because you are professional in front of the woman and then you have a laugh in the staff room don't you, and it's so difficult because

the students shouldn't really be listening to all the stuff that goes on, should they?

(M10/T1/H)

Despite what mentors thought, students were acutely aware of professional behaviours.

The way you behave with the women. Your behaviour with other members of staff, how you interact with each other.

(S22/T2/G5)

What you do and say when you're out of the room as well is a big thing. I mean if you go out and start saying terrible things about the woman or a family that you're caring for, that's not very professional … is it?

(S17/T1/G5)

The comments in the PADs support the view that students were expected to and usually managed to embody professional standards. Most mentors wrote on almost every opportunity about students' professionalism.

A naturally professional approach.

(S41/T3/G9)

Presents herself well, always professional in her manner.

(S39/T2/G8)

Always professional in her attitude.

(S4/T1/G1)

While the official discourse for mentors was to establish and maintain professional boundaries and contribute to the development of an environment in which effective practice is fostered (NMC, 2008). The new standards (NMC, 2018) continue to reinforce the expectation that effective practice learning is essential for all students. However, many mentors recognised they did not always uphold this competence. They rationalised the stressful environment and trusting one another in certain times and places with these less than acceptable professional behaviours. Goffman's (1959) on-stage metaphor can be applied to places where midwives considered they were upholding the professional values, which is in front of the women. However, when midwives were off-stage, in the coffee room, for instance, their behaviour was not always as professional as it should have been. The students seemed to understand that they always had to behave professionally; there was no off-stage area for them as their character and manner were always under scrutiny.

4.3 Progress of learning

The ability to acquire and develop midwifery knowledge, in the first year, especially, seemed dependent upon a continuous relationship with one mentor.

I hadn't connected with anybody because I didn't have a mentor at all, so I felt like, and I still feel I'm sort of six months behind all the time because of that experience.

(S33/T1/G8)

The impact of no relationship is seen in the language the student used. S33 felt she had missed half of her learning opportunities during the year (she says she is 6 months behind after 14 months as a student). Another student, who was seven months further on in her education (21 months) articulated:

It depends on your experience of practice particularly on whether you've got one or two mentors which you work with regularly and you've built up a good relationship with, or whether you're being passed from pillar to post to a new person every couple of days who doesn't know what you're capable of, isn't comfortable necessarily letting you develop your practice as smoothly as you would if you've got that continuity.

(S19/T3/G5)

A lack of continuity was detrimental to the students' learning as the student must convince the mentor to let them practise skills. S19 recognised this limited her opportunity to select and practise the skills she wanted to develop. The hierarchy and control between the student and mentor are stronger when the mentor does not know the student well enough; she 'isn't comfortable necessarily letting you develop'. With continuity of mentorship, the student and mentor can work together, and the selection, pacing, and sequencing of the student's practice is often discussed to enable to student to progress 'smoothly' rather than in a repetitive fashion. This was corroborated by the Hughes and Fraser (2011) study, discussed earlier, where continuity of mentor is seen as an issue for all students, but particularly first and third years. In the final year, mentors' confidence to enable students to work independently depended on the amount of time they had spent with the students (Hughes and Fraser, 2011).

In the interview with M9, I asked about the sequencing and pacing of practice.

So, who then decides whether they [the student] take part in the booking interview or all of the booking interview? (SCM).

Well, with that example, I will discuss it with the student first to see what they feel confident to do. If they say that no they don't want to do any of it, and I feel actually you've shown me skills that you could do this (M9/T3/C).

Yes (SCM).

I would then just move them on a tiny bit. I would say why don't you just do this and this and then I'll do the rest, so when they feel comfortable doing that, just let them do a bit more. You do get students who are a lot more confident than other students. If you had a student that perhaps said I could do it all and perhaps [I] felt that actually we haven't covered a lot of this then I would ultimately be the one to say, 'Well no, we'll do [it] this way'. So, I think there is still that definite line there, but I think it's better to do it in partnership with the student rather than telling them what to do (M9/T3/C).

The definite line is the structural relation between M9 and the student. Initially, M9 masked the hierarchy between her and the student, by asking the student what they wanted to do. This is weak framing (F–). However, if the student did not appear confident enough, and M9 felt the student could undertake the activity, she encouraged them to take part. The framing altered (F+). Similarly, if the student was too confident, the mentor again controls the student's participation (F+). Either way, M9 knows she is in the hierarchical position, but she prefers not to use this control, thus weak framing (F–).

I did not ask M2 about the pacing of learning in clinical practice, she told me spontaneously.

> I like to have, at the start of placement a sort of interview ... above what we do on paper ... and then at the end of the placement I just like to have a chat with them [students] after the paperwork to see where they are. I usually like to get them to write a bit of reflection on their practice as well ... I'll get them to do something else, a bit of homework for instance, if they are weak on some aspect.
>
> (M2/T3/H)

My interpretation of this pedagogic relationship is that the mentor likes to be in control of student learning (F+). However, during the interview she seemed to relax her initial authority (F–) when she talked about the importance of the first meeting with a student, 'It has to be outlined what it is the student expects and what it is the mentor expects and then find a common ground in-between' (M2/T3/H). Here, again, depending on the student–mentor relationship, the pedagogic relation alters between strong or weaker framing strengths.

Evidence from the students' PADs showed a range of midwifery knowledge and skills acquired in the first year. It also suggested students who learnt quickly were valued.

> Has progressed excellently in first placement. Confident, quickly able to perform abdominal palpation and blood pressure under indirect supervision. Communicates well with women. Needing no prompting. Well done. I look forward to working with her again.
>
> (S41/T3 first community placement)

> Student has progressed exceptionally well with regards to her initial community placement. She is competent at performing basic care, i.e. blood pressure and urinalysis. She always confirms with the mentor any information/care that she is unsure of and therefore is a safe practitioner at this stage of her training. I have found her to be willing to undertake tasks requested in an

appropriate way to ensure women do not feel uncomfortable or embarrassed that she is training, i.e. VE.

(S35/T2 first placement community)

Most students had learnt some basic clinical skills, and examples of these were explicitly stated in the entries. Once students were proficient at the basic clinical skills, little feedback was offered on these in the PAD. Different clinical skills which are considered interventions, for instance, amniotomy or induction of labour, were generally not documented until the final year or months of students' education. Thus, one can hypothesise, basic midwifery skills are an essential requirement that all students must learn rapidly in the clinical environment; perhaps so they can take part in the workload. This means the pacing of these skills is initially strong. This changes as less emphasis is placed on the pace of acquisition of the more advanced clinical skills or interventions, especially by mentors. Students became increasingly concerned about their lack of ability and confidence in these as qualification approached. Areas for the development of fundamental skills, such as vaginal examinations and abdominal palpation, were noted in third-year students' feedback; thus, an inference is made that a basic understanding rather than a mastery is sufficient until the student is just about to qualify, when the significance of these skills increased.

Elements of relationship development were also interpreted from the PAD, such as mentor pleasure at the opportunity to work with the student again (S41 above). Similarly, the second extract (S35 above) shows strong framing as the mentor directs the student to undertake clinical tasks, while the first student needs no prompting.

Here, student-led learning is documented.

Student has identified areas of practice to improve upon and taken steps to achieve this. i.e. leading clinics which improved confidence considerably. Always watchful and observant and keen to improve in all areas. Able to trust the student will come for help and explanation. Always putting women's feelings and situations first to find ways to help them.

(S1/T2 end-point community interview second placement of first-year placement)

If students recognise what is expected of them, they have a greater opportunity of selecting learning opportunities to show their knowledge.

4.3.1 Acquiring 'hard' clinical skills

Several times in the interviews, students and mentors presented phlebotomy, taking blood, or venepuncture, as an example of how learning occurred in theory and practice. The process of learning this skill, it seemed, was more visible than learning other types of practice knowledge. While these skills were presented in

Chapter 3, here the transmission and acquisition of them, including the choice and pace of learning is offered.

A good mentor will not have a big build-up to it, so we'll see with this one and then she'll make the decision after she's asked the woman and then tell you, this time you're going to do it (S36/T2/G8).

So, if there is a big build-up for a long period of time where you've got to worry about it, that's worse for you? (SCM).

Yes, it makes you nervous (S34/T1/G8).

Yes, that's what happened with my first mentor, and it was horrible (S36/T2/G8).

I had quite a wait to do venepuncture because my mentor didn't want me to do it on somebody who was scared and so everyone was scared so I didn't get to do it for the whole of my first placement and then it started to become a thing that I need to do as I'm going to worry about it now. Then I got put with a different mentor ... and she went, 'Well I'll let you look at the woman's veins and if you're happy, then just go ahead and do it'. I did, and she was doing her paperwork while I was doing it, and she wasn't all over me, and afterwards I just wanted to go 'Yes! Did everybody see that? I did that all on my own', cause my [first] mentor would undo the tourniquet, or she'd pass me the cotton wool, and I wanted to do it, all of it on my own, so that I knew I could. (S34/T1/G8)

Here two different mentor styles affect the students' ability to learn. S36 starts by saying her preferred learning style is for the mentor to have explicit control, strong framing, for the mentor to show her one procedure and then for her to be directed to undertake the next one. She labels the mentor as 'good' because the expectations are clear, and the mentor has not allowed the student to become too anxious about the task.

However, S34 described strong framing and her experience where her first mentor took control of the choice of the student's learning opportunities by using women's fears to mask the mentor's apparent anxiety. The second mentor not only enabled the student to learn but also enabled the student to decide, depending on the woman's veins, whether she was confident to continue. The locus of control was with the student, thus weak framing. The mentor did not directly observe the student in this skill acquisition; however, the student wanted recognition of her achievement. The 'help' from the first midwife undermined the student's skill development and confidence.

While S34 wanted her mentor to see her performance, not all students feel close observation from their midwife is beneficial.

I was doing some venepuncture at an antenatal clinic, and I was being watched very closely, and I couldn't do it ... I don't have any problem with that, and I'm absolutely fine, and I'm fine with my midwifery mentor watching me, no problem but with other things sometimes like palpation things I want them there so even though they're not standing over you watching but that you've got that reassurance…. so, it depends on the situation and on who is that is watching you and what their approach is, whether you feel they are there to support and help you or to see if you're doing it wrong.

(S19/T3/G5)

The student articulated the balance between being watched and being supported; sometimes, she wanted reassurance and her mentor's presence at other times she felt scrutinised.

A mentor who believed in the student's ability was more empowering than one who took over, as this next student shows:

I went to take blood, and I don't know if I missed the vein, something went wrong, and I was like all ready for like a certain midwife who would have taken over and done it, but my mentor was just like got it all ready and asked if she was happy for me to try again and the woman was like yeah that's fine, and she was like do it again. I was like OK and first time, done it, and she was like 'see'. A different person would have taken over, and I would have left there being like 'Oh I've forgotten how to take blood', whereas I left there being like yeah. It must have been a weird vein, and I did it. I wasn't expecting her to give me a second go, but the woman was like 'No, that's fine', and the mentor told me to go for it. And she was like I know you can do it, and I was like oh, so yeah.

(S39/T2/G9)

These examples show how the relationship with the mentor can affect students' access to and development of skills.

4.4 Busy clinical environments and overstretched mentors

Mentors recognised the challenge of supporting students in an environment that was overstretched.

Just that there is a huge demand on mentors at the moment in practice and you know …. there's big issues with staffing shifts, being changed at the last minute and we allocate students to a named mentor, and then they might find that the off duty's been changed of their mentor and they [students] can't necessarily change at the last minute.

(M1/T3/H)

Mentors, especially hospital-based staff, expressed the difficulty of teaching first-year students, especially when they were busy or unwell.

There seems to be a lot of people [mentors] that don't have any students, I mean I'm all for having students but just occasionally, a couple of shifts where you work independently. Like I say especially when you've got first years it's like for six or seven weeks every shift with you, and yeah, it's a lot … I said to Kay [pseudonym] I need to be backed off at the moment because I'm not feeling as great and they're [students are] not going to benefit from me, but I was told there's no other mentor.

(M3/T3/H)

It is quite time-consuming because you want to show them [first years]. With a third year, they are helping you with the paperwork, with a first-year you're having talk through the whole way through.

(M10/T1/H)

Yeah everything takes ten times longer.

(M11/T1/H)

And when you've got more than one woman, it is because it is really, busy, which is really difficult because you just want to get on with it.

(M10/T1/H)

When it's busy, and I am a bit of a perfectionist, I know that, so sometimes I find it hard to actually let someone take over. I am aware of that though, so I think it's about, I'm quite happy when a student says I see you do that a couple of times, I'd like to do it.

(M7/T2/H)

Mentors from each Trust discussed the implications of student learning needs and the impact of this on their workload. Most mentors recognised they prioritised the work before student learning. First-year students were considered more work as they were time-consuming. The absence of the word teaching was noted in most mentor interviews and can be interpreted to mean this activity was less significant than completing the work.

Community mentors in Fisher and Webb's (2008) two-stage correlational study also explained the difficulty of mentoring first-year students. Having to go back to a basic level and being exhausted by constant questions was recognised as a challenge to midwives (Fisher and Webb, 2008). At the time, students in the Fisher and Webb (2008) study spent the whole first year on the community, which may explain the mentors' perspectives. Six mentors took part in a focus group to determine 15 needs of mentors. Three further mentor needs were found in a literature review, including adequate staffing and frequent shifts with students (Fisher and Webb, 2008). All 18 needs were included in a questionnaire distributed to 82 eligible mentors, of which 57 returned the survey. Most of the mentors (n=47) were nurses prior to becoming midwives, and the majority worked in a hospital (n=40) (Fisher and Webb, 2008). These demographics may have influenced the mentors' need for support, and the negative undertones expressed about first-year direct-entry students. This included having a break from them and considering young, direct entry students harder to mentor than the registered nurses (Fisher and Webb, 2008). Three-year students with life experience were generally viewed more positively as they helped with the workload (Fisher and Webb, 2008).

In my study, all the mentors above worked in the hospital setting. They too found first years harder to mentor especially when they were busy. It is interesting to note though that all the above mentors were direct entry students themselves.

Students too recognised mentors competing responsibilities within the busy environment.

> The mentors are very pressured aren't they, they are still doing their full-time job, and they've got you as an addition, and I think because of how busy the wards are, and you know if there's sickness on that day and the actual input that they're afforded to give you there is no protected time you know.
>
> (S16/T1/G4S)

> I know obviously, they're [mentors are] doing their job, and the wards are busy, and we're like a little extra, even though it shouldn't be like that but it kind of is, isn't it?
>
> (S39/T2/G9)

The findings resonate with Kroll et al.'s (2009) mixed-methods study exploring students clinical experience on a postnatal ward, where two main themes affected the learning: the culture and the mentorship. Due to insufficient mentors, students often felt they were working independently, and the culture of getting the work done was prioritised above the students learning needs.

There was one area of midwifery practice where the environment seemed more conducive to student's learning: the community.

> I think mentors in the community as well they see more of your practice and your communication everything like that because they are with you all the time, whereas in the hospital the midwives tend to leave you with the women on your own for periods of time to see if you build your confidence up on your own, but they don't actually see what you're doing.
>
> (S24/T1/G6)

In the community, the student and mentor are in close physical proximity most of the day; this closeness enables the mentor to see more of the student's practice. Sanderling University students tended to work with one specific community mentor, returning to them each year. One of the barriers to effective mentorship, which was the lack of continuity, was removed, so the student could focus on learning from that mentor. The community environment seemed more receptive to students in the Hughes and Fraser (2011) study. Students in Kroll et al.'s (2009) study also found they were better supported in the community setting, and they too preferred the one-to-one teaching in this environment. The possible interpretations made were how busy the hospital staff were and how much harder this was for mentors (Kroll et al., 2009; Hughes and Fraser, 2011). However, community mentors in Fisher and Webb's (2008) study, especially those who had been qualified for more than 15 years, found time to support students on the three-year programme rather intense. The balance between student and mentor needs is clearly not a local issue.

Lack of time in clinical practice was a feature of almost all the mentorship research (Nettleton and Bray, 200; Armstrong, 2010; Longworth, 2013; Rooke, 2014; Moran and Banks, 2016). Nettleton and Bray's (2008) research of nursing, midwifery, and medical mentors and mentees used two forms of data collection, questionnaires and interviews to conceptualise positive and negative men-tor—mentee relationships. The questionnaire was pilot tested, which increases its reliability. However, typically low response rates from mentors (13–26%) were received, with greater percentages from mentees (39–60%). The findings between the participants were separated so the midwifery responses can be identi-fied; however, no midwives were interviewed (Nettleton and Bray, 2008).

All mentors thought their role had little recognition in the workplace. Most of the midwifery respondents (64% n=20) considered they needed more time for their role and a few also requested more training (12% n=4). Mentees desired will-ing mentors, yet most of the nurses interviewed explained they became mentors because they were expected to, instead of choosing the role. Students in my research also perceived mentor reluctance and a need for further mentor education and time.

In an evaluation survey of the NMC (2008) *Standards*, 114 new sign-off men-tors, 37 mentorship students, and 13 nursing and midwifery lecturers were posi-tive about the introduction of the sign-off mentor's role (Rooke, 2014). The sign-off role is a requirement set by the NMC. In nursing the sign-off mentor is allocated for students' final placements to authorise entry onto the professional register; however, in midwifery education, all students should be assessed by a mentor with this extra level of responsibility during their course. Rooke (2014) expressed concerns about the support available for sign-off mentors. The three-phase study looked initially for views from sign-off mentors, then registrants completing the mentorship course, and finally lecturers (Rooke, 2014). The response rates were 95%, 45%, and 28%, respectively, with those in the sign-off role responding in greater numbers. This may have influenced the findings, which the author acknowledged. While the survey included views of midwives, these were not separated in the findings. However, workload and lack of time were still considered the greatest challenges to the mentoring role (Rooke, 2014).

Thus, there are several tensions which impede the quality of teaching and learning in clinical practice: busy hospital environments, a lack of mentors, time, and workloads. This should be balanced with the learning needs of students.

4.5 Pedagogical relationships and practice learning

Despite a diversity of aims and research methodologies used in the literature to support this chapter, a common theme was the need for a positive relationship between the student and mentor; it was essential for practice learning (Moran and Banks, 2016; Longworth, 2013; Hughes and Fraser, 2011; Fisher and Webb, 2008; Fraser et al., 2013).

The process of acquisition within a framing relation can be depicted as:

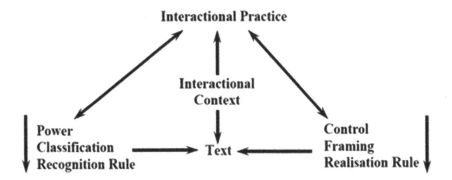

Figure 4.1 Transmission context.

Figure 4.1 explains the concepts previously introduced and the relationships between them. Classification, whether strong or weak, orientates students to recognising a specific context (or not) from another. Recognising the context is essential for students to demonstrate a legitimate 'text' or appropriate performance (as explained in Chapter 3). The recognition rule refers to power relations. However, recognition alone is not sufficient to realise the appropriate 'text'. If students do not possess the realisation rule, they will be unable to perform or practice appropriately. Framing regulates the specific realisation rule which enables meanings to be put together to create the legitimate text. The amount of control a student has over the selection, sequence, and pace of the acquisition of their learning will affect their ability to demonstrate a specific text. The interactional practice is shaped by classification and framing within the interactional context. The text is anything that attracts evaluation, from how the student moves to what they say, and is produced as a response to classification and framing and interactional practice.

Initially, I was surprised by the lack of content in the interviews about the knowledge necessary for clinical midwifery practice. However, using Bernstein's theory, the relationship between students and mentors is more pertinent, and this is what helps or hinders access to specialised knowledge. The literature used in this chapter can also be related to Bernstein's relational practices or framing strengths. For instance, Bluff and Holloway (2008) found that the prescriptive midwives tended to be older with more experience. They often had the status and position of sister (or senior midwife), and this legitimated their positional power. Students in their study, and mine, noticed their lower status and imitated the prescriptive midwives' practice to avoid conflict.

The flexible midwives tended to be younger and lower in the hierarchy (Bluff and Holloway, 2008). Most of the midwives interviewed in my research reflected this younger, more junior demographic. They were also considered 'good' mentors by the students; however, they still differed with respect to framing strengths and, depending on the interaction with a particular student, encouraged or discouraged certain student behaviours. Some of the student experiences with more controlling mentors may have been from older midwives with higher positions; however, I did not ask this question. Certainly, one of the negative student comments about inappropriate behaviour was directed at a senior midwife, although her age was not mentioned. This can be understood when Bernstein says strong framing is positional and weak framing is personal. The position of the senior midwife gave her status, whereas the younger midwives tended to appear friendlier and closer to the students.

Features of strong and weak hierarchy and mentor control were also clear in the Hughes and Fraser (2011) study. The qualities, expectations and experience of a mentor, their ability to role model and the relationship, all affected the students' learning experience. There was agreement that a good mentor was approachable, instiled confidence, advocated for women, and used evidence to inform their practice (Hughes and Fraser, 2011); like the flexible midwives (Bluff and Holloway, 2008). Conversely, mentors who undermined students, did not explain their practice or were resistant to having their practice questioned were considered less effective (Hughes and Fraser, 2011; Bluff and Holloway, 2008). A welcoming relationship with a mentor was valued by the students, while more controlling mentors were viewed as less helpful. The problem of some mentors expecting students to do everything, and others limiting learning experiences was also expressed (Hughes and Fraser, 2011). The student and mentor relationships in my study also differed with respect to this hierarchy.

Role modelling was one way that mentors showed students what was needed (Finnerty and Collington, 2013; Hughes and Fraser, 2011). However, not all students perceived this as a method of teaching. Bernstein's (2000) visible and invisible pedagogies can be used to explain this phenomenon. A visible pedagogy is one where the classification and framing are strong while an invisible pedagogy had weak classification and framing. If the practice knowledge being taught was venepuncture, already established as strongly classified knowledge, and the mentor showed and explained the skill to the student and then used a fading technique, the student would be more likely to recognise this as a teaching strategy. If however, the mentor role modelled excellent communication skills, discussed as weakly classified in the earlier chapter, and then asked the student to offer information to another woman, the student may not perceive this as teaching. The manner of the mentor as well as the subject affected some students' ability to 'see' the clinical learning. This is implied in the first theme in McIntosh, et al.'s (2013) study: where students thought they taught themselves midwifery.

In any transmission of knowledge, something must happen first, and something will then follow this is progression. Pacing is the expected rate of acquisition, how much the student must learn in each amount of time (Bernstein, 2000). There is quite a lot of variation between midwifery students regarding experiences gained and skill development. Most students had three years to complete all the requirements, with the minority on the shortened 78-week course. Some skills, such as venepuncture, seemed fundamental to midwifery practice and early acquisition of this skill was essential for student achievement and progress. It was almost a rite of passage. Other skills were introduced later in the students' education.

Most students in my study, and other research, thought they progressed further with continuity of mentorship (Hughes and Fraser, 2011; Fraser et al., 2013). The need for students to learn their mentors' preferences is documented, and when students knew these they could progress in their development. Once students understood the preferences of their mentor, they were better placed to assert *their* opinions and authority, and this enabled their learning needs to be met.

Several types of practices between individual mentors were noted but also between different areas. The community seemed a more receptive environment than the hospital setting, from the student perspective (Hughes and Fraser, 2011; Kroll et al., 2009). It was preferred as it offered more access to the mentor (Kroll et al., 2009). However, some mentors, especially those with 15 years or more experience, found the longer student placement in the community intense and this could affect the quality of the mentoring relationship (Fisher and Webb, 2008). The busy pace of practice was a barrier to learning (Armstrong, 2010), especially in the hospital (Hughes and Fraser, 2011). Here, students sometimes felt they were working independently (Kroll et al., 2009).

Some midwives demonstrated unprofessional behaviours. These were sometimes rationalised by mentors due to the stress of the workload or environment. Mentors generally felt they needed support to undertake their role (Moran and Banks, 2016; Rooke, 2014; Fisher and Webb, 2008) and the lack of time to teach was frequently identified as a barrier to practice learning (Moran and Banks, 2016; Longworth, 2013; Kroll et al., 2009; Nettleton and Bray, 2008). When midwifery lecturers taught students clinical skills in the university setting (Longworth, 2013; Fraser et al., 2013), more time and feedback was afforded than the practice setting (Longworth, 2013). However, a small majority of students considered that clinical practice provided a better opportunity to learn skills, despite some students having to work hard to access these opportunities (Longworth, 2013).

The practice environment is much more nuanced than past studies may have shown. The environment seems to vary according to the context of practice, mentors' perception of the importance of practical knowledge acquisition, and students' experience. Diverse types of learners and pathways into midwifery have implications for the learning process. For instance, the students who entered the midwifery practice arena with no previous experience, healthcare knowledge, or earlier nursing qualifications had differing orientations to the meaning and learning in clinical practice. For some groups, the learning was visible through observation and an explanation of care, for others, this was invisible and limited. Some students could affect the relationship positively between themselves and their mentor; others had limited power or knowledge of how to influence this. All these aspects affected the learning in clinical practice.

Since this research was conducted, the NMC has published new standards which support practice learning (NMC, 2018). While the role of the mentor no longer exists, the functions of this role to support and assess students in practice remain. However, instead of one registrant inhabiting both roles, the NMC (2018) have separated these functions and two new practice roles now exist: the practice supervisor and the practice assessor. The NMC (2018) states that there is a need for sufficient coordination and continuity of support and supervision of students to ensure safe and effective learning experiences. So some of the aspects students felt necessary remain.

The practice supervisor should act as a role model, enable the student to meet their proficiencies, provide feedback, and support the student to participate in the practice learning (NMC, 2018). As already stated above, midwives do this to varying degrees in their role as mentors. The new practice assessor role was created due to concerns that mentors were failing to fail students, and their objectivity was clouded by the close working relationship with students. In order for practice assessors to make a judgement about a student's practice or performance, the NMC (2018) has stated that they should periodically observe the student across environments in order to inform decisions for assessment (NMC, 2018). The new standards (NMC, 2018) are considered in the final chapter under the change of code section in further detail.

Bibliography

Armstrong, N., (2010). Clinical mentors' influence on student midwives practice. *British Journal of Midwifery*, 18(2), pp. 114–123.

Bernstein, B., (1990). *Class, Codes and Control Volume VI The Structuring of Pedagogic Discourse*. London: Routledge Taylor and Francis Group.

Bernstein, B., (2000). *Pedagogy, Symbolic Control and Identity Theory, Research, Critique*. 2nd ed. Oxford: Rowman and Littlefield Publishing Group inc.

Bluff, R. & Holloway, I., (2008). The efficacy of midwifery role models. *Midwifery*, 24, pp. 301–309.

Finnerty, G. & Collington, V., (2013). Practical coaching by mentors: Student midwives' perceptions. *Nurse Education in Practice*, 13, pp. 573–577.

Fisher, M. & Webb, C., (2008). What do midwifery mentors need? Priorities and impact of experience and qualification. *Learning in Health and Social Care*, 8(1), pp. 33–46.

Fraser, D., Avis, M. & Mallik, M., (2013). The MINT project – An evaluation of the impact of midwife teachers on the outcomes of pre-registration midwifery education in the UK. *Midwifery*, 29, pp. 86–94.

Goffman, E., (1959). *Presentation of Self in Everyday Life*. New York: Doubleday Anchor.

Holland (2010). Fitness for practice in nursing and midwifery education in Scotland, United Kingdom. Journal of Clinical Nursing, 19, pp. 461–469.

Hughes, A. J. & Fraser, D. M., (2011). There are guiding hands, and there are controlling hands': Student midwives experience of mentorship in the UK. *Midwifery*, 27(4), pp. 477–483.

Kroll, D., Ahmed, S. & Lyne, M., (2009). Student midwives' experiences of hospital-based postnatal care. *British Journal of Midwifery*, 17(11), pp. 690–697.

Longworth, M., (2013). An exploration of the perceived factors that affect the learning and transfer of skills taught to student midwives. *Midwifery*, 29, pp. 831–837.

McIntosh, T., Fraser, D., Stephen, N. & Avis, M., (2013). Final year students perceptions of learning to be a midwife in six British universities. *Nurse Education Today*, 33, pp. 1179–1183.

Moran, M. & Banks, D., (2016). An exploration of the value of the role of the mentor and mentoring in midwifery. *Nurse Education Today*, 40, pp. 52–56.

Nettleton, P. & Bray, L., (2008). Current mentorship schemes might be doing our students a disservice. *Nurse Education in Practice*, 8, pp. 205–212.

NMC, (2008). *Standards to Support Learning and Assessment in Practice*. London: Nursing and Midwifery Council.

NMC, (2018). *Standards for Student Supervision and Assessment*. London: NMC.

Rooke, N., (2014). An evaluation of nursing and midwifery sign off mentors, new mentors and nurse lecturers' understanding of the sign off mentor role. *Nurse Education in Practice*, 14, pp. 43–48.

5   The evaluation of learning

This chapter will consider the evaluation of learning in the clinical area. The evaluation of learning is a judgement about whether students have met the criteria (Bernstein, 2000). The criteria can be explicit and specific or implicit, multiple, and diverse. The students were evaluated by their mentors qualitatively on each long (four weeks or more) placement, as well as quantitatively at the end of each practice module.

The three-year students usually completed nine or ten long placements during their course while the 78-week students had six or seven. Qualitative feedback, from the mentor about the students' performance, was scheduled at the mid-point and end of each placement. The practice modules lasted one year, the exception to this was the first 78-week module which was six months. The quantitative grade was derived from 20 criteria, based on four domains of practice outlined by the NMC (2009, p.21). Students and mentors used the 20 criteria to evaluate the students' performance. The final grade is awarded after a discussion of the students' and mentors' grades during a tripartite meeting with the student, mentor, and lecturer. Thus, the criteria are multiple and diverse.

This chapter draws on student practice grades and practice assessment documentation to consider the evaluation of learning. Most students received high grades for practice, despite the differences in students' ability to recognise and realise the rules of practice, differences in mentor expectation, areas of practice, and student–mentor relationships. The face-to-face interaction between the student and mentor, a social process, meant some students had the ability to influence the grade they were awarded.

The timeliness of feedback from long placements, the negotiation of grades between the student and mentor, and where the final grade was obtained are all discussed. During the case study, the grading tool was amended twice. The first change sped up the grading process and was well received. The second change, however, caused more discussion as students thought it negatively changed their practice grades. The reasons and implications of the changes to the grading tool is offered in Section 5.2.

5.1 Student practice grades

One hundred and twenty-four students started the two programmes from February 2009 to February 2013. Ninety-three students were enrolled on the three-year programme (0209 n=17, 0210 n=17, 0211 n=21, 0212 n=22, and 0213 n=16) and thirty-one on the shorter 78-week course (0209S n=7, 0210S–0213S n=6). Twelve students left the three-year course early in their studies. Two students from other universities transferred into this programme during year 2. This meant there were (93–12+2=) 83 separate students' grades considered in this analysis. The grades from the first year of the three-year programme do not count towards the final degree classification, as the university had a 24/76 ratio for calculating classifications derived from the second- and third-year's work. Thus, the 83 students' grades from the second and third year are considered, as these contribute to their final degree classification. Only one student left the 78-week course prior to her first practice grade. Consequently, 30 separate students' grades are included, as they all contributed towards the final degree classification.

On the three-year course, 75% (n=114) of the students were awarded first-class practice grades (see Table 5.1). A further 11% (n=17) were awarded 2:1 grades; collectively, this is 86% of the practice grades at 2:1 and above. On the 78-week course, 75% (n=43) received first-class practice grades with 14% (n=8) awarded a 2:1 (see Table 5.2). Collectively this is 89% of the practice grades at the higher levels. The pattern of practice grades between the two programmes is therefore similar and concurs with other published literature presented in Section 1.4.

Few students were referred in practice (n=7 on the three-year programme and n=3 on the 78-week programme). One student was failed and withdrawn due to practice failure from each programme. The other eight students passed the practice module following a further opportunity. Their grades were capped at 3 (40%). These findings concur with a retrospective survey of 27 UK universities (52% response rate) which compared the referral rate for student nurses theoretical and practice assessments (Hunt et al., 2012). The number of students who were referred and withdrawn due to practice failure ranged from 0–4.25%, which amounted to just one student in some universities (Hunt et al., 2012). Students who were referred in practice usually passed at a next attempt (79.5%) (Hunt et al., 2012). In nursing, students were more likely to be failed in practice in their second year (Hunt et al., 2012). At Sanderling University, most referrals for midwifery practice were in the final year. These cases will be discussed in detail in the following chapter.

The grades suggest that most students are performing very well and that only a few are not at the expected level. This indicates that mentors can differentiate between students who are succeeding in midwifery from those that are not. However, according to Bernstein (2000), a graded performance should show differences between students. It is an assessment for stratifying how well the student has met the criteria. As there is limited stratification of student performances, I suggest that mentors have assessed competence.

The focus of a competence assessment is not upon a gradable performance, rather on similarities between students. The students are judged by mentors to share common competences and by the end of the course are eligible to enter the professional register. Therefore, the act of grading symbolises authorisation from the mentor that the student is performing as expected rather than an objective measurement of their practice. This demonstrates a mismatch between reality and the standard to grade practice (NMC, 2009).

Table 5.1 Three-year students' grades from years 2 and 3

Number of grading episodes	Left	Refer	3	2:2	2:1	1-	1=	1+
151	7 so no grade awarded	9 (7 students) 8.4% of students	6 (all second attempts)	5	17 (11%)	28 (19%)	43 (28%)	43 (28%)
							75%	
					86%			

Table 5.2 78-week students' grades

Number of grading episodes	Left	Refer	3-	2:2	2:1	1-	1=	1+
57	7 so no grade awarded	4 (3 students) 10% of students	2 (both 2nd attempts)	8 14%	7 12%		25 44%	11 19%
						75% of grades awarded		
				89%				

Tables 5.1 and 5.2 also show the spread of first-degree classifications. At Sanderling University, there were three first-class bands: 1–, 1=, and 1+, which represent 70–79%, 80–89%, and 90–100%, respectively. Most students on both courses are awarded grades of 80% or more for practice (56% and 63%, respectively). This was noted in the literature too (Seldomridge and Walsh, 2006; Scanlan and Care, 2004; Walsh and Seldomridge, 2005) with nearly all practice grades at the higher end of the spectrum.

5.2 The grading tools

The practice grades presented in Tables 5.1 and 5.2 are not directly comparable as the Sanderling University grading tool changed twice over the five years of the curriculum and this case study. Sanderling University may not be unique in amending its grading tool. Briscoe et al. (2006), in their study of 129 US medical schools, noted that the majority (57.8%) of evaluation tools had been recently created or revised. Many were only in use for 1–4 years (Briscoe et al., 2006).

Table 5.3 Example of one statement and marks available from the January 2009 grading
tool

20–16	15–11	10–6	5–0	*Mark awarded by*		
				Student	*Mentor*	*Agreed*
Effective midwifery practice						
Excellent links made between knowledge and practice	Very good links made between knowledge and practice	Good links made between knowledge and practice	Limited links made between knowledge and practice			

At Sanderling, the 20 statements did not change; however, the marks available
for each were amended (see Table 5.3).

The midwifery lecturers agreed to make some amendments to the grading tool
after reflecting on the first year of grading practice; collectively, they had been
present for 48 student tripartite assessments (Chenery-Morris, 2011). The time
necessary for the students and mentors to negotiate a grade was generally one
hour, although some lecturers had been present for longer than this. The lecturers received some negative comments from practice partners about the length of
time needed to complete the grading process, especially with a student who was
progressing as expected.

In physiotherapy education, 78% of 41 clinical educators considered the time
taken to complete the students' clinical evaluation was unacceptable (Murphy
et al., 2014). The mean time for their assessment was 80 minutes with a standard deviation of 53 minutes (Murphy et al., 2014). The introduction of a new
grading tool reduced this to 23 minutes (SD 13), and no educators found this
unacceptable (Murphy et al., 2014). Time pressure for clinical grading is also a
notable finding in the comprehensive systematic review by Gray and Donaldson
(2009a). The lack of time for practitioners means the assessment feels like a task-
orientated burden rather than an integral element for student learning (Gray and
Donaldson, 2009a).

In addition to the time pressure, the likelihood of students or mentors being
able to differentiate between such discrete measures of performance was also considered unrealistic (Wolff, 2007). The difference one point constituted to the
grade was negligible on the Sanderling University 2009 grading tool (20 statements × 20 points available = 400 points; 1/400 × 100 = 0.25%). Students and
mentors usually negotiated small increases or decreases in the final grade, which
hardly affected the outcome; more on this will be presented in Section 5.3.1. It
was also noted that mentors and students usually chose the same boxes, either in
the very good or exceptional range.

In their review, Gray and Donaldson (2009a) found a wide range of grading
tools with scales from four descriptors to 40 and a visual analogue scale ranging

Table 5.4 Example of one statement and marks available from January 2011 grading tool

4	3	2	1	Mark awarded by		
				Student	Mentor	Agreed
Professional and ethical practice						
Excellent ability to express personal feelings and identify learning from experience	Very good ability to express personal feelings and identify learning from experience	Good ability to express personal feelings and identify learning from experience	Support required to express feelings and identify learning from experience			

from 0 to 100. Hence, the midwifery lecturing team decided the same descriptors would be used with one grade for each box, rather than a range in the grades awarded for each criterion (see Table 5.4). This gave a score of up to 80 points instead of 400. The change was approved through the usual university processes. This was intended to speed up the grading process and reduce the number of discrete measures of performance.

The first student and mentor interviews undertaken in June 2011, just after the grading tool was amended, were mostly positive.

> The new numbering 1–4 on the tripartite assessment is much better.
>
> (S5/T1/G2)

> It's greatly improved
>
> (S6/T2/G2)

> This is quicker, the new way. I think you know you can still prompt discussion on things but not as easily as you would with the old tool.
>
> (M2/T3/H)

However, the last comment reflected some hesitation from M2, that the older tool enabled greater discussion of student development.

The expected *minor* change affected the grades awarded; resulted in even higher practice grades and in some cases students were awarded 100%. From the literature, practice grade ranges from 65 to 100% (Plakht et al., 2013) and 69 to 100% (Hiller et al., 2016) are documented from 124 and 547 students, respectively. Therefore, awarding such high practice grades is known. However, the reduction in the amount of discussion meant the students received less verbal

Table 5.5 Example of one statement from amendment 2 May 2012

1–3	4	5	6	7–10	Mark awarded by		
					Student	Mentor	Agreed
Developing the individual midwife and others							
Requires support to identify appropriate learning opportunities	Seeks out learning opportunities with some encouragement	Actively engaged in learning within the practice environment	Proactively identifies and engages in learning opportunities within the practice environment	Exceptional ability to enhance learning at every opportunity			

feedback on their practice. For these two reasons, a further change was made to the grading tool in May 2012 (see Table 5.5).

After much discussion, the midwifery team chose the word exceptional for the first-class boundary (7–10), in an attempt to ameliorate the number of high grades. A range of grades was considered beneficial, especially when students were at either end of the spectrum. This enabled students and mentors to award a first but not the 98 or 100% seen with the earlier tool. It also offered more discussion for mentors to show students how they could increase their grade from seven to nine or how they were under-performing with their practice with the lower grades.

5.2.1 Reactions to the 2012 grading tool change

Two main complaints were made about the final grading tool: the terminology and its potential effect on student grades, and the range of grades in the first-class boundary.

> The paperwork had changed, and I felt that it was very unfair, the paperwork, cause all of a sudden there was a massive jump where it's 7, it's graded 1–10 and 7–10 is excellent. So, you can't seem to get an excellent or outstanding. It is a massive word itself, and they [mentors] are so reluctant to give it to you and then the next grade down is such a big jump from that to excellent.
>
> (S30/T1/G7)

> To get 70% you've got to be outstanding or something and I wouldn't say that I am outstanding at anything, whatever it is, but you know sometimes I feel that well actually yeah, I could get 7 out of 10 in that, but I would never say that I am outstanding. So, to me, the words and the numbers don't compare.
>
> (S29/T2/G7)

> To get even a 7 you have to be exceptional. And a 7 out of 10 to me is not that good.
>
> (M12/T1/C)

> Yes, it's that exceptional word, and if you want to be able to have the opportunity to get a 7 if you're really good and it's one of those things especially when you go into practice, and I think this is for everyone who goes into practice, I don't think there's anyone who doesn't try their 100% and really works hard in practice.
>
> (S40/T2/G9)

The final quote from S40 implied she wanted the grade awarded for effort as opposed to accomplishment, for trying her best instead of her performance.

This 78-week student discussed the range of grades for the top marks.

One thing I remember with the grading tool it's hard and quite different from exceptional you must have, it's from 7–10, and I think it's a wide range to be, I don't know exactly, subjective. Because maybe you can be 4, 5, and 6 are a little bit more in the middle of the grading and 7 to 10 is four numbers, just for exceptional. It doesn't seem fair?

(S47/T1/G11S)

Her thoughts were echoed by a mentor and lecturer.

It is not easy, especially with the system. Like, we were saying this last time that it says 7 to 10. How can I grade 7 to 10 if the criteria are the same?

(M14/T2/H)

The mentors and the students had difficulty understanding what the difference between exemplary at 7 and exemplary at 10, and compared that to the other boxes in the midrange where you had one box for one banding.

(L1/T1)

The reason there was more discussion about this change, perhaps, is that the tool reduced some student's grades.

I don't think it helped that the sheets were changed because I know I dropped 20%. I know it didn't worry me because I thought the first year perhaps was really high, that could have put some people off to quit because that could be disheartening (S38/T1/G9).

So, you think that by dropping that much it could really affect how you see your progress in midwifery? (SCM).

It could have done, but it didn't for me and also it was a different mentor (S38/T1/G9).

Here, S38 is still awarded a first; her 20% reduction was from a mark in the 90s to the 70s. Acknowledging that it was a different mentor mitigated against some of her disappointment. The implication of her words is that the grade really does matter to the student, and a low practice grade may affect their identity and commitment to the profession.

The word 'exceptional' was considered to be a barrier for some mentors and students. However, when the final grades were examined, most students still received over 70% for their practice (see Tables 5.1 and 5.2). Therefore, what the participants believed about the word 'exceptional' and how grading was enacted did not align.

5.2.2 *Interference with the grading process*

The lecturer's presence was a reoccurring theme across the interviews. Some students liked their personal tutor hearing how well they had progressed in practice.

Conversely, negative comments about two lecturers' behaviour during the assessments were expressed. The students were respectful and did not mention the lecturers' names. This student started by imitating the lecturer's words:

> You are looking at 5–6's in your first year, 7–8 in your second year, and 9–10 in your third year. And that would be where she'd expect you to be. Now having spoken to other people that may not have the same tutor, that's not how they've been graded, and that makes me worried about what my grade is. I know it's obviously OK, but it is going to, it's lower than where I want it to be … My mentor was constantly calling me a second or third year because she thought my knowledge and things were really good. You feel really good, but my percentage didn't reflect that because she was doing it how she'd been told to do it. I mean it was fine, but it wasn't up there with the firsts which is where I'd prefer it to be.
>
> (S41/T2/G9)

The mentor thought the student's performance was at a level higher than her status and year of experience, yet this was not the grade she received. The authority of the lecturer, it seemed, had influenced the student's practice grade. The mismatch between the verbal feedback given by the mentor in practice and practice grade is also documented in Heaslip and Scammell's (2012) research. When mentors (n=112) were asked whether their feedback corresponded with the grade, 89% (n=100) thought it did. However, only 60% (n=65 of 107) of the nursing students agreed (Heaslip and Scammell, 2012). The difference in belief was attributed to mentors preferring to give positive feedback rather than constructive criticism. Heaslip and Scammell (2012) do not say if there were any other influences in their study; in my research, the presence of a lecturer added another layer of interpretation to awarding practice grades.

The unwelcome interference was echoed by 78-week students.

> And the grading … I felt it was really unfair.
>
> (S51/T1/G11S)

> Yeah, it was from the beginning, just saying that we should be between 5 and 6, so that was always interfering with the marks that we were given because she was like saying the criteria it's not changing it but using the tool in a different way than other mentors or other teachers.
>
> (S47/T1/G11S)

> I think that the knock-on effect of that was the situation I had was that my mentor in practice thought that was the way that it was supposed to be done that we should be graded a slightly lower level to allow room for improvement that's what she had been told by colleagues of hers and in fact when it came to do the tripartite there was a big difference between what I had graded myself and what she assessed me as. But luckily my personal tutor was

able to put her straight, so we were able to sort of meet in the middle, but still I wonder if she hadn't been given that sort of conflicting information, whether that mark might have been higher, ultimately.

(S50/T1/G11S)

When S50's personal tutor was present at the tripartite, she explained to the mentor that all marks were available to grade the student's progress, but S50 was still concerned that the mentor had been unduly influenced by the previous information and this may have negatively affected S50's final grade.

One of the lecturers admitted how she tried to make the practice grades align to a standard deviation curve, rather than the dichotomous pattern.

I explained it to the students and the mentors … in any form of assessment you should get a standard deviation curve and to me that's what that grid now does, it's that you've got a lower end and a higher-end, but the bulk should be in those three boxes in the middle … I kind of used that as my preliminary … I don't think you're going to be in the top and bottom end too much, but I am not sure that I wasn't using it to try and control, to make the tool do what we wanted it to do. So, I felt that I wanted them to really, really justify if they'd given themselves 7, 8, I gave them a much harder time in justifying why they thought they were exemplary, than probably if they'd had given themselves a 6. So, I am not sure that I used the tool equitably … and I think that conflicts and I was wrestling with when I was using it with the guidance that we'd written, which says 'All marks are available for all students, whatever their year'.

(L1/T1)

The inconsistent use of the grading tool by the university staff caused confusion and was a source of dissatisfaction for some students.

But surely, we should have some sort of instructions for that because no one has a clue. When you go in there, without being rude, the tutors don't have a clue because you got all different information from each tutor. The mentors don't have a clue and the students don't have a clue, so when, I know of one student that got marked, and she got marked as a midwife. Do you know what I mean?

(S30/T1/G7)

This student's sense of frustration is palpable; there is so much interpretation of the grading process that it seems no one has the 'correct' solution.

There were a few positive comments about the May 2012 change, however none from students.

I personally feel that the latest version of the grading tool that we are using is much more effective in terms of applying an appropriate grade to the student which isn't elevated unnecessarily … the fact that we now have a fifth box has meant that it is far more discerning and that's been complemented further by the explanations to the mentors as to what equating it to the degree classifications has really, really emphasised what an exemplary student looks like.

(L4/T2)

While this lecturer considered the tool more discriminating, the grades do not show this trend, with almost all students still receiving a first for practice regardless of the tool used.

5.2.3 Not receiving a first for practice

For the students who did not get a first though, their grade had the potential to affect their self-esteem.

Yeah, you don't want to give yourself a 4, and then they give you a 3, and then you feel like you're really stupid. I think it depends whether you are on the higher side or the lower side, because I didn't get the best mark on mine and everybody else got like 80 or 90%, and I got like I don't know 69 or 68 or something, and I came out feeling like the biggest pile of crap in the world, so when you get higher marks, it's easy.

(S17/T1/G5)

If you got that in an essay, you'd be over the moon.

(S19/T3/G5)

Yes, but in practice, because everybody else gets great marks if you get a bad mark, you feel really bad whereas if you get a bad mark in an essay it's not so bad.

(S17/T1/G5)

The small cohorts at Sanderling University facilitated most students sharing their grades, whether these were theory or practice grades. Knowing and voicing that a practice grade was not as high as other students had detrimental effects on students, as S17 and others also confirmed. One student declined to be in the group interview, explaining she was not happy with her grade and would be upset if she talked about it for the research. Others were more able to share their experiences, even if they were negative.

I came out of there really disappointed. Areas where I know that I was really good at, I felt was lowered and between the certain person and my mentor, it was suggested that we shouldn't be sort of 70–80%, that we should be for our level just coming in to it. That we should be looking at 50 and 60s, that had a massive impact on the marking.

(S51/T1/G11S)

This mature, qualified nurse cried during the interview, possibly due to the frustration and impact of her lower practice grade. Accordingly, for students, there was a tangible sense of emotion built into their practice grades. For some, the emotion was positive and reassuring as it was associated with a high practice grade, yet for others it was demoralising and felt unfair.

With different opinions in the lecturing team and in practice, grading was problematic. This concurs with the literature (Scammell et al. 2007; Gray and Donaldson, 2009a). Scammell et al.'s (2007) qualitative study of students, mentors, and lecturers' experiences of a newly implemented grading tool found confusion and misunderstanding and different interpretations of the assessment document despite their attempts at mentor preparation. Inadequate knowledge about the grading tool impacted upon its use. Students said mentors were unable to award the high practice grades they wanted (Scammell et al., 2007). While it was not clear where the perception originated, there were reports that university-based staff wanted students to produce more evidence for the higher grades. This had the potential to undermine the mentors' confidence and authority in grading (Scammell et al., 2007). It also undermines students confidence in the process.

The aim of the systematic literature review undertaken by Gray and Donaldson (2009a) was to explore the issues with grading practice, including reliability and validity. Validity was considered in terms of the grading tool and process of grading. Both the tool and the process were criticised by Sanderling students. Inter-rater reliability was also documented as problematic with inconsistent interpretation of the criteria (Gray and Donaldson, 2009a). Consequently, Gray and Donaldson (2009a) determined the usefulness, reliability, validity, and effectiveness of grading of practice was still to be proven.

5.3 Impression management

To make a favourable impression on mentors, students often had to suppress their feelings about the uncertainty of their practice grade. Much of the anxiety about grading came from the need to self-assess.

On mine I put two stroke three.

(S23/T2/G6)

Oh, do you?

(S25/T1/G6)

Because I'm not really sure where I fall, and obviously, I fall in the middle, but when I'm doing my tripartite you know a decision needs to be made which one you're going to be ... I find that really, really hard ... I feel in the middle ... I think that's where the five box just needs to come into play.

(S23/T2/G6)

Students across separate groups were fearful of being overly confident with their grades.

> Yes, I don't want to, not that I'm big-headed anyway, but I just feel like even if I feel 'oh I can do this', but I don't want them to feel that I'm putting myself high when I'm not, I just don't want them to look at me and like yeah whatever … If you give yourself a 3 and you're like I'm sure I can do that even with supervision but you still sometimes feel maybe I should put myself as a 2 so they can look at that, and it's their mark at the end of the day, isn't it … I think if your mentor thinks that you're big-headed, then they'll probably mark you down anyway, I think.
>
> (S18/T3/G5)

S18 shows how difficult it was to self-assess her grade and defers to the authority of her mentor 'it's their mark'. A reoccurring theme across the student interviews was how students projected their identity in the grading process, if this was above or below what their mentor considered proper there could be repercussions.

> And you read them and think well I think I'm this but if I put that, am I going to get marked down because they'll think, I think I'm great.
>
> (S34/T1/G8)

> Like big-headed.
>
> (S37/T1/G8)

> Or if I put, so if I put the next one down, they're not going to mark me up from that because I put that. So, you feel like it's a bit of a game.
>
> (S34/T1/G8)

> You don't want to go too low because then they'll think you've got a lot of don't know what word I'm looking for.
>
> (S37/T1/G8)

> Not a lot of confidence.
>
> (S33/T1/G8)

> Yeah, confidence and stuff, and then they'll ask a million more questions.
>
> (S37/T1/G8)

> It's a little bit of a mind game as to what to put.
>
> (S34/T1/G8)

This impression management was especially important in grading themselves (Goffman, 1959). When an individual is in the immediate presence of other people, he or she will seek to control the impression that others form of him or her to achieve their goal (Hivid Jacobson and Kristiansen, 2015). The other participant in the encounter will attempt to form an impression of who and what the individual is. The student's performance or 'front' is the attitude, presence, and expressions used to construct a certain image of who he or she is. These students thought a mentor would reduce their grade for being overconfident and be subject to further scrutiny if not confident enough. This was a valid thought reiterated by mentors.

> A good student who in my eyes wants to learn, has set objectives, is keen to work, works well within the team, doesn't you know, works effectively independently but also knows when to not [to] independently but with guidance, but not someone whose quite cocky, we get the odd one that comes through that you think, 'Well you keep saying things like that, you're going to really annoy people', but they are sort of my good students, all-round.
>
> (M3/T3/H)

Similarly, at another Trust:

> You hear your colleagues, don't you? If they are too loud, they are too cocky, if they are too quiet, they're too shy. You've got a have a happy medium, and it's very difficult to get like that.
>
> (M10/T1/H)

> You get a student come in, in the first year and you're like 'I don't like her, she's a bit cocky'. I think she knows it all.
>
> (M11/T1/H)

Acceptable student behaviour throughout their time in practice needed careful consideration of impression management, which many students were aware of.

The following vignettes show the strength of student feeling and how they tried to manage a more favourable impression of themselves in practice.

> In the first year I absolutely hated it, I didn't know what to say, I didn't know what to do, the mentor didn't know what to do … I found it really uncomfortable saying well I have been really proactive, and I've been really enthusiastic I think I deserve'
>
> (S4/T1/G1)

S4's words, show how her feelings were suppressed to enact the role of the student, or the role she assumed she needed to project, one of enthusiasm. Enthusiasm, as with effort earlier, is not one of the explicit grading criteria; however, it probably contributes to an overall positive mentor evaluation of the student.

A student who visibly lacked confidence in their self-assessed grade the first time and tried to show more confidence in their self-assessed grade the next time explained her experience.

We went into it not really understanding the process, was asked to complete a form that I didn't understand very well and it kind of leant itself to under-estimating yourself because you didn't want to look as though you knew everything ... people were urging me to have more confidence and to put better grades. By the second year, I was thinking of, using that information and the next time I would, I would say I think I am doing better, only to be told well actually you're not there quite yet. It was the same people but at different times.

(S26/T1/G6)

Even though the same people were involved in the grading process and encouraged S26 to be more confident, her self-assessed grade was apparently too high at the end of the second year. However, this was one of the first students to say her personal tutor influenced the grading process.

Mentors thought students tended to offer a lower grade than they deserved; perhaps this was part of the game. The students left room for the mentor to raise their grade, as they were the authority.

Yes, they [students] probably underestimated their abilities a bit. But I think everybody does that anyway. Because you don't want to look like the bees' knees when even though you are, you don't put it on paper, do you, so. But I did for her.

(M3/T3/H)

I interpret the reason some mentors raise the students' grades as a feature of their relationship with the student; it reassures the student that they have been accepted and can increase their confidence in practice.

Say you got 85 in an essay then you'd be like wow, that's crazy, publishable, whatever. Whereas if you got 85 in a tripartite then you'd obviously come out with better marks than I think I would have got from the theory side of things and it gives you more confidence, but at the same time it feels a bit like, well it's easier to get higher marks in some of those in the tripartite.

(S19/T3/G5)

Even knowing it is easier to achieve a high practice grade, this student expresses how her confidence is increased by a high grade. Another student found the tripartite meeting offered more feedback on her performance than the earlier qualitative mid and endpoint meetings. The presence of the lecturer appears to have influenced the mentor's performance.

I like the tripartite; I like clarification that I'm doing things right and that I'm OK and so I find that in the tripartite you get that, I get that. Whereas sometimes some people will be like in practice, so you know that was really good, or that wasn't so good or whatever but in the tripartite the mentor actually really goes into more detail which is what I like about it.

(S1/T2/G1)

This student was clearly articulating the need for more in-depth feedback from the mentor and the tripartite grading process offered that. She altered her language from 'you' get that to 'I get that', to show how other students might not agree, but for her it was positive. Many of the other student group discussions corroborated this student's experience, that they lacked detailed feedback on their performance in practice. However, this comment also suggests some sort of objectivity in the grading process, with the opinion that practice can be 'right' as opposed to a subjective enacted encounter.

For some students, the grading process was of immense value.

The only thing that I would say that up until that point [the tripartite] about how she was going to go, I hadn't had an awful lot of feedback up until that point, so I was really worried and nervous about what she was going to say, and then it turned out that it was fine, so I always assumed that things were OK, but she might have said before now if it wasn't going to be good, but I still didn't know because up until that point she hadn't really said what she thought. On the first year that was a very first time that they [say] how good you were doing or how bad you were doing.

(S26/T1/G6)

This student was unsure about her practice performance. She assumed she was showing the right skills, but the lack of feedback caused her uncertainty. For her, as with S1, the tripartite grading discussion was in more depth than their earlier experiences of feedback.

S44 explained why she would expect a first for practice.

I'd have been very disappointed if I hadn't got a first, over 70% on that [practice]. Because I felt from the feedback that I'd had and the interviews that I'd had and from everything that happened in the three years, nothing had even been pulled up that I needed to improve or change apart from developing my skills and knowledge.

(S44/T1/G10)

I think I would have been [disappointed], I did find it hard; it got easier but the self-grading thing. I found I probably lacked confidence compared to you [talking to S44] and I did under mark myself but gradually over the years that improved.

(S45/T1/G10)

When students receive positive feedback from practice a logical conclusion is that their performance calls for a high grade. S44 repeated the notion that she under-graded her performance and attributed this to a lack of confidence. The reason students' and mentors' grades are higher at the end of their training could be attributed to the increased confidence that comes with time enacting a role, professional enculturation. However, it could be due to the weak boundary between the student and mentor at the end of the course. In occupational therapy education, student grades had a statistically significant increase in the second and third years (Roden, 2016). A total of 593 student grades were analysed with a rise of 1% in each year. Reasons for the increase included students modelling their behaviour to fit the criteria, and they become more skilled at this each year. In addition, students respond to constructive criticism to improve their performance (Roden, 2016). However, as already noted, not all midwifery students thought they received much feedback, and few discussed constructive criticisms, so this element of learning may be missing from practice.

5.3.1 Student-mentor negotiation of grades

To follow up on the students' discussions, the 26 Practice Assessment Documents were analysed to see the range of students' self-assigned and mentors' grades and process of negotiation (Appendix 11 for the full data set).

From the seven 78-week PADs, 14 summative grades were awarded. Twelve of these were on the original tool, and two on the 2011 version.

Table 5.6 shows that mentors awarded slightly higher grades than the students on Tool 1 on both assessments. The grades for Tool 2, albeit only two students, shows the student self-assessed grade was 1 point higher than their mentors. On 10 of 14 occasions (71%), the mentor elevated the student's grades, on 3 occasions, the grade was reduced (7%). One PAD has identical grades for the student and mentor for each of the 20 descriptors; therefore, it suggests the grades were awarded jointly instead of independently. In the first six months, the differences between student self-assessed and agreed grades range from 10 points fewer to 77 points more out of 400 (a 2.5% reduction and 19% gain). More often, the mentor raised the student's grade by 5%. For the final grade, one student's grade was lowered by 2/80 points (2.5%). The greatest rise was 10%.

Table 5.6 78-week student negotiated grades

Analysis	Grade at 6 months	Grade at the end of training	
Student self-assessed grades ranged from	Tool 1 (n=7) 61–82%	Tool 1 (n=5) 78–88%	Tool 2 (n=2) 94–96%
Mentor grades	Tool 1 70–89%	Tool 1 78–90%	Tool 2 94–95%
Agreed grades	Tool 1 70–85%	Tool 1 78–90%	Tool 2 94–95%

Table 5.7 Three-year student grade analysis

Analysis	Year 1	Year 2	Year 3
Students	Tool 1 (n=2) 312–340/400=78–85% Tool 2 (n=12) 60–75/80=75–94% Tool 3 (n=2) 105–142/200=52–71%	Tool 2 (n=5) 69–78/80=86–96% Tool 3 (n=14) 90–167/200=45–84%	Tool 2 (n=2) 70–79/80=88–99% Tool 3 (n=17) 127–196/200=63–98%
Mentors	Tool 1 339–342/400=84–85% Tool 2 63–80/80=79–100% Tool 3 121–142/200=60%–71%	Tool 2 70–80/80=88–100% Tool 3 101–196/200=50–98%	Tool 2 80/80=100% Tool 3 125–196/200=62–98%
Agreed	60–98%	50–98%	62–100%

The three-year cohort used all three of the grading tools (n=2, n=19, and n=33, respectively).

Table 5.7 displays the three-year student–mentor negotiated grades. The difference in the Tool 1 grades, for two students was –1/400 to +4/400 from student self-assessed to mentor-agreed grades, which is negligible. With Tool 2 the difference ranged from –4/80 to +14/80 (a decrease of 5% and an increase of 17%). However, most students were only awarded one or two extra points. Tool 3 grades ranged from –14/200 to +53/200 (a decrease of 7% and an increase of 26%). The majority were raised by approximately 10%. Even when student grades were reduced, they were often still in the first-class range. However, Tool 3 did cause the greatest variation and this, as well as the slightly lower grades, may have contributed to the students' frustration with this iteration. Mentors raised the student's grades on 38 occasions (67% 38/57 occasions) and lowered eight grades (14%). The remaining 19% suggest the grading process was completed together, or the data was missing.

The number of times mentors raised the grades was similar between the two courses (71 and 67%); however, there was a slightly higher rate of reductions (14%) in the three-year course, compared to (7%) in the 78-week course. The mentors may have been able to exert greater control over the grades of the three-year students compared to the 78-week students' grades due to the classificatory value between students on one course or the other (Bernstein, 2000). The category of three-year students compared to 78-week students can, according to Bernstein, have a different space in which to develop their unique identity. If the classification between the two types of students is strong, they are distinct kinds of students. If the classification is weak, they are similar. Section 4.2.1 discussed the difference between students on the two courses. Mentors articulated a difference between students on the two courses; thus, the 78-week students had a different identity from the three-year students. The identity of the 78-week students as already qualified nurses may have affected whether mentors felt able to control these students' self-assessed grades as often in relation to the three-year students' grades.

In the literature, presented in Section 1.2.1, when 124 nursing students self-assessed their practice, it was accurate 60% of the time (Plakht et al., 2013). Accuracy was measured by a student grade within –5 to +5% of the mentor's grade (Plakht et al., 2013). Over-estimation was a gap of more than 5% and under-estimation less than 5%. When this same measurement is applied to the three-year midwifery student/mentor grades, 40% (18/45) were accurate. The missing data and identical student and mentor grades were not counted. Most students 54% (24/45) under-assessed their performance with 6% (3/45) over-assessing their performance. The 78-week student grades were accurate 76% of the time (10/13). Fewer students 3/13 (23%) under-assessed their performance, and no students over-graded themselves.

The mentors reduced the grades occasionally in both cohorts, but most of these were within 5%; therefore, using Plakht et al.'s (2013) accuracy measurement the student grades would be classified as correct. This means the number of students over-assessing their performance is far fewer in midwifery students at Sanderling University than nursing. However, this is a small sample, and the grading tools changed. This analysis does support the student and several mentors' feelings that students tend to under-grade themselves and that mentors tend to raise the students' grade; this seems to happen more often with the three-year students.

The amount that mentors raised or reduced students' grades was minimal; thus, this was a symbolic act. Accordingly, depending on whether the grade was increased or reduced, there was a positive or negative effect on the student. The students who undertook the grading jointly with their mentor may have been those who were less confident of their self-assessment abilities or ones who preferred not to be subject to the process of self-disclosure. They may also have had a more relaxed relationship with their mentor, as this student explains.

> Think in terms of the grading, I know we've all had a little discussion about this it is sort of the case of that you want to get on well with your mentor because you feel like it will affect your grade.
>
> (S14/T2/G4S)

5.3.2 Mentor confidence in grading

Impression management was as important for mentors as students. Students evaluated their mentor's ability and confidence in the grading process.

> I think also depends on how long you have worked for them for doesn't it … Cause some of them are really confident of that you're definitely a

15 and others say well you could be, sometimes you're this, and sometimes you're that.

(S2/T1/G1)

The factors that seem to affect the grading process were the length of time a student and mentor worked together, and the mentor's confidence.

It all depends on your mentor, doesn't it? (S5/T1/G2).

It definitely depends on your mentor some will just quite happily agree with what you've written (S8/T3/G2).

Sign you off, yeah (S5/T1/G2).

Whereas others will think about it and actually tell you no, I think you're higher than this because or you're a bit lower than this because. That is much more helpful (S8/T3/G2).

These students found specific feedback on the strengths and weaknesses of their performance helpful. This was when the criteria rules were made explicit to them by the mentor (Bernstein, 1990). S8 suggested she received constructive criticism. However, the use of 'a bit' implies the positives outweighed the negative comments from her mentor or the mentor framed the negative feedback in this way.

The importance of mentor preparation and confidence in their role is featured in the literature (Gray and Donaldson, 2009a; Heaslip and Scammell, 2012; Scammell et al., 2007). While most mentors, 64.3% (n=72), were confident to grade practice there was a disparity in the qualitative and quantitative feedback offered to students (Heaslip and Scammell, 2012). The authors postulated this discrepancy could be due to a lack of confidence in mentors offering constructive feedback or in students recognising they were receiving feedback. However, if the feedback is only provided at the end of a placement it does not enable the student to improve their practice. Plakht et al. (2013) found student development was improved by high-quality discussions on areas for development rather than focussing on the positive. In my work, students also respected the mentor more who offered a discussion rather than a 'you're fine' response. This was a feature of implicit criterial rules, and the student was unaware of the criteria they had to meet (Bernstein, 1990).

By 2012 grading of practice had been operationalised for 3 years, but there was still a sense that mentors were not familiar with the process.

I think that they find it quite difficult, they're not familiar, well they say they're not familiar with the practice grading. They don't understand how it works; they have to have it explained to them all the time (S20/T2/G5).
Who explains it? (SCM).
Me and then it kind of feels like you don't want to lead them into making a conclusion but when they go, 'What does this bit mean?' and your kind of, you want to say well this is when I am doing this, that and the other, so you

are really telling them well … whereas really, they should be familiar with it themselves and make the decision off their own judgement (S20/T2/G5).

This student explained how she interpreted the criteria for the mentor, and in doing so she understood the potential to influence the mentor. S20 was not sure whether the mentors were not familiar with the paperwork, or they were testing the student to see how they explained it. What she seemed to want was the mentor to decide how well she was practising and offer that feedback independently.

Not all students agreed with this:

I think it depends on the mentor, some of them are familiar, and some aren't, and some are confident in, you know, might not have seen it before but are confident to read the guidance in our PAD documents and draw their own conclusions from that. I think it's always the mentors I've worked with it's always been (a) consultative process it's always 'Are you happy with what I've written here?' And 'If I sign you off at this level are you happy with this?' … I find it very hard to grade, to grade myself in what I think is, you know, reliably accurate.

(S19/T3/G5)

Here S19, who has an earlier degree, managed to separate the ongoing assessment of progress from the grading process. The relation between the ongoing assessment and grading was not always made distinct in the student's discussions, which is understandable as the two assessments are related. This student may have found the process consultative because she was always explicit in her communication and articulated the problem or care decision succinctly.

While some students were sceptical that mentors understood the grading criteria, several mentors explained how they used it explicitly.

I think it's good, I think because you can look at their criteria and say and give them examples of why they are doing it rather than just saying [to] them it's fine. I think it's good and I think that it's really good for people that aren't doing so well because you can then show them the criteria for what the good grades are, the high grades and say you need to be doing this as well as, you can't just do the bare minimum and go and deliver someone's baby, you need to be giving it the whole, you know.

(M1/T3/H)

Similarly, this student understood how the criteria were used explicitly.

You are face-to-face with your mentor, and she's got to justify what she's given you, as much as we've got to justify what we think we've achieving, and she doesn't want to look bad to us as we don't want to look bad to her or not meeting our targets.

(S23/T2/G6)

This section shows that grading practice is a social process. The student, mentor, and lecturer at the tripartite meeting were engaged in a process of mutual surveillance, testing out each other's beliefs and responses, and negotiating interactions. Students saw mentor confidence and lecturer inconsistencies, and some could influence the grade awarded.

In my field notes, I documented student–mentor interactions. Some students and mentors came prepared to the meeting, like the student above explained, with notes on why they deserved higher or lower grades and examples from practice. This strategy often produced a greater depth of discussion and the prepared party's ability to influence the grade. Another student, who protested how much she hated the grading process, pushed the PAD away from her towards her mentor when her mentor reduced the student's self-assessed grade. This act of frustration or disappointment disassociated her from the awarded grade; it was the mentor's responsibility. The manner of her action was symbolic of dissatisfaction in the grade, but she was unable to explain why she deserved her self-awarded grade. Mentors anticipated the reaction of the students. If students managed favourable impressions of themselves, it often led to a higher practice grade.

5.4 Placement-specific grades

Several students thought their practice grades were placement-specific and that one practice grade each year was not sufficient as it did not reflect all their practice experiences.

> I think with the tripartite at the end of your year, if you are just with a community mentor you might be competent in community, but you might fall to bits on Labour Suite … Not that I did, but I know that I had a good relationship with my community mentor and did well, but my CDS mentor might have thought differently (S36/T2/G8).
>
> That's why you can have them both, can't you? If you've done both placements, you can have a mentor from both, and they can meet in the middle (S37/T1/G8).
>
> But you're not going to do that, are you? (S34/T1/G8).

S36 was careful to preserve an image of competence in front of her peers. She offered an example of a student being competent in one area but not another, then quickly qualified that was not her experience. The student explained that different areas of practice have different competencies, and being graded at the end of the year is not sufficient to encompass all that is midwifery. While some students did manage to get both community and hospital mentors together for the final grade, there were several reasons why students would not do this. First, the practical issue of arranging a meeting with the lecturer and two mentors was difficult. Next, the student is more likely to choose the mentor they felt most confident with or, the one they knew the longest or had most recently, so the assessment was as contemporaneous as possible.

One student discussed the problem with one summative practice assessment.

> That's what happened to me on my second one because I had a community midwife come to my tripartite and she was grading me as if I was in the community and I'd downgraded myself as I was referring to myself as I am in the hospital, and she's never seen me in the hospital, so she found it quite difficult to see where I was coming from because she sees me as someone that's confident at doing something, but I feel in hospital … I lose a lot of my confidence.
>
> (S23/T2/G6)

While S23 did not explain her loss of confidence, when she introduced herself at the beginning of the interview, she acknowledged: 'I was probably very unconfident about the course, nothing in my previous life had prepared me for this … and probably lack of confidence was my biggest thing and assertiveness, which is changing'. S23 may have developed confidence in the community placement where the student and mentor work closely most of the time, where the schedule for the day is likely to be predictable (visits, clinics etc.), and there are fewer if any emergency events. Although, she admitted that in the hospital she lost confidence, and this affected her self-assessed grade.

When something is missing in a students' performance, such as confidence, it is attributed to explicit criterial rules, and the student is aware of the omission (Bernstein, 1990). Bernstein explained that in each encounter or evaluation of a student's performance there are two discourses: the regulative and instructional. 'The pedagogic discourse embeds a discourse of competence (instructional) into a discourse of social order (regulative) in such a way that the latter always dominates' (Bernstein, 1990, p. 183). The rules of social order, relation, and identity are embedded in the evaluation of the student, and when S23 lacks confidence in a certain area, it is because this is the necessary requirement to perform legitimately in this place. When the criteria are explicit, the performance of the student can be graded, but the evaluation of the students' performance is only relevant in that specific context (Bernstein, 1990). Therefore, to be meaningful to the student and reflect their performance in each area, every placement should be graded.

5.4.1 *Timeliness of feedback on student progress in practice*

During the group interviews, there was a consensus that students did not get sufficient formal feedback.

> The start is usually at the start, mid-point is usually at the beginning of the last week because finally they've [mentors have] realised hang on a minute we haven't done the mid one, and you're going to ask me for an end one in a few days, so that's usually when that happens and the end one happens on the end date, or you have to come back a few days later for it to be done.
>
> (S37/T1/G8)

Here, the students are slightly sarcastic about the feedback they should receive. They explained that despite the curriculum having allocated times for meetings this rarely happened. Other student groups supported this.

> In terms of getting time with people [mentors] to do the meetings, I don't know about you, but I always found that very difficult to pin people down, when it's busy, there's no time.

> (S45/T1/G10)

To quantify when feedback was received, I developed a RAG rating score based on the timing of the feedback. The dates of the handwritten feedback to students in their PADs were cross-referenced to the dates they were allocated to the placement area. Green meant all meetings occurred as scheduled. The first meeting was within the first week of placement with mid and endpoint meetings evenly spaced. Amber was a delay of one meeting (greater than one week for the first), or one of the meetings was not completed. Often the first and mid-point interview or mid and end-point were undertaken/dated together. Red was where the meeting occurred after the placement had ended. This was rated red because it was an inconvenience to the student and not pedagogically sound. The student had to return to the placement and had usually begun their next placement before they had received feedback from their last. Consequently, they started a new placement without firm knowledge of how well they had performed or what they needed to develop next (See Appendix 12 for RAG colour coded placements for three-year and 78-week students).

Table 5.8 represents 165 long placement reviews for 19 three-year student midwives. Table 5.9 illustrates the analysis of all students RAG-rated feedback from each area. The largest proportion (43%) of the student feedback was received from CDS midwives, with slightly less received from the community (36%). Nevertheless, when the two placement areas are compared, the ability of midwives to adhere to the planned feedback varied. On CDS, there were 71 evaluations in total with 36% of the feedback rated red, 34% green, and 30% amber. This meant students had almost an equal chance of receiving feedback as planned, late, or after the placement had finished. When this is compared to the community, the number of green-rated evaluations was greater, with 61% adhering to the curriculum.

Table 5.8 RAG rating for three-year students by placement area

Placement	Green	Amber	Red	Total
CDS	24	21	26	71
Community	36	12	11	59
Ward	7	6	5	18
MLBU	7	9	1	17
Total	74	48	43	**165**

Table 5.9 Analysis of 19 three-year students' feedback

Placement	Green	Amber	Red	Total
CDS	24/71=34%	21/71=30%	26/71=36%	71/165=43%
Community	36/59=61%	12/59=20%	11/59=19%	59=36%
Ward	7/18=40%	6/18=33%	5/18=27%	18=11%
MLBU	7/17=41%	9/17=53%	1/17=6%	17=10%
Total	74=45%	48=29%	43=26%	165

Reasons for this increased rate of adherence to the planned curriculum in the community may be attributed to better workload planning. In a busy hospital environment, planning time for mentors and students to meet is dependent on each shifts' workload. There is a belief that the hospital's workload is less predictable. The interpretation of this finding is that the relative value of the scheduled meetings was especially low in the hospital. Formal feedback meetings were not prioritised, or able to be prioritised, by mentors in all practice areas. I suggest it could also be a feature of the increased face-to-face contact between the student and mentor in the community that was lacking in the hospital.

The 78-week students had slightly better green-rated placements overall (Table 5.10), with 53% (compared to 45% in the three-year programme). However, there was still some variation between placements. Most community placements (79%) were rated green (see Table 5.11). Mentors in the hospital, on the ward and CDS, were least able to offer prompt feedback. Table 5.12 shows both programmes. Less than half of the students (47%) received feedback as planned. One in four student placements (25%) were rated red. Compliance with practice feedback was discussed in relation to medical education (Hiller et al. 2016; Lawson et al. 2016) in Section 1.1.3. However, there was no documented evidence in the nursing and midwifery literature of this phenomenon and its potential effect on student learning and outcomes.

Some students appeared to have better 'luck' or could perhaps negotiate the schedule of their meetings (Appendix 12). Five of the 26 students managed to have only amber or green placements. So even for students who might be most

Table 5.10 RAG rating for 78-week students by placement area

Placement	Green	Amber	Red	Total
CDS	8	6	5	19
Community	11	2	1	14
Ward	3	3	3	9
MLBU	3	1	1	5
Total	25	12	10	47

Table 5.11 Analysis of seven 78-week students' feedback

Area	Green	Amber	Red	Total
CDS	8/19=**42%**	6/19=**32%**	5/19=**26%**	19/47=**40%**
Community	11/14=**79%**	2/14=**14%**	1/14=**7%**	14/47=**30%**
Ward	3/9=**33%**	3/9=**33%**	3/9=**33%**	9/47=**19%**
MLBU	3/5=**60%**	1/5=**20%**	1/5=**20%**	5/47=**11%**
Total	25/47=**53%**	12/47=**26%**	10/47=**21%**	47

able to negotiate their placement evaluations, the ones which were delayed or combined were in the hospital environment. Other students were either less fortunate or unable to negotiate or organise feedback from their mentor; these students had far more red evaluations than amber or green Table 5.11.

Two students' PAD showed difficulties with placement evaluations. S31/T3, despite being on the three-year programme, only had seven long placements in all. Of these, five were rated red, one was amber (community), and one green (community). Sh/T1 on the 78-week programme had four red evaluations; all in the hospital. The only student from the sample this had a profound effect on was S31. It nearly affected her ability to qualify; her case is explored in Chapter 6.

Some individual mentors though, regardless of where they worked, hospital or community, were noted in the PAD to either fall into a likely to be a green category or likely to be a red category. Mentors who agreed to be part of the study, M13/T1/H and M10/T1/H, regularly managed to complete the paperwork as planned despite working on CDS, but yet another CDS mentor at another Trust seemed to be less able to supply prompt feedback. Similarly, one mentor in the community always seemed to require students to complete their paperwork after their placement, sometimes a month later.

Table 5.12 Both programmes together

Area	Green	Amber	Red	Total
CDS	32	27	31	90
Community	47	14	12	73
Ward	10	9	8	27
MLBU	10	10	2	22
Total	99/212=47%	60/212=28%	53/212=25%	212

During the mentor and student interviews, reasons for conducting the meetings late were discussed. S14/T2/G4S was reluctant to have her first interview too soon and did not particularly value the meetings.

I like a week to settle in, and then I've a week before my second interview and then two weeks before my final interview … If I've got them [mentors]

> working with me and I have time to do the interviews in the first place, three
> interviews in four weeks is not, it seems a bit stupid really to be honest.
>
> (S14/T2/G4S)

As a 78-week student with a master's degree already, she may not have felt
the need for such frequent feedback. However, other students wanted the reassurance they were meeting expectations as some were uncertain about their
progress.

When asked if assessments were conducted in work time, many students and
mentors reported that there was no time for this to happen within the working day.

> My mentor last year did come in on her day off basically. Bless her (S5/T1/G2).
>
> They shouldn't have to (S7/T1/G2).
>
> No, they probably shouldn't have to but then they don't get time (S5/T1/G2).

> Were the assessments carried out in work time (SCM)?
>
> Hell no (S9/T2/G3).
>
> True, we never get them done in work time (S10/T3/G3).
>
> No, I've always had to arrange them out of work. Some mentors preferred to
> conduct these meetings in their own time (S9/T2/G3).

> I'd rather do it in my own time because, you know it's really difficult to
> arrange a time with someone whether it's just for the grading or anything to
> do with the student's paperwork.
>
> (M1/T3/H)

Therefore, some of the red-rated interviews may have been a mentor or student's
preference rather than necessity. One student revealed,

> There were times we could have done our meetings and she [mentor] was
> doing other things, not midwifery, that I allowed to go on because I thought
> fair enough, I know my book will be signed in the end.
>
> (S13/T2/G4S)

The inference made by the student is that she permitted the mentor to avoid the
paperwork, knowing it would be completed eventually. However, I suggest the
student did not have the authority to negotiate a meeting, despite it being necessary for her development and a requirement of the curriculum. Other students
recognised they were a potential burden for mentors.

> I always find it really hard to get a mentor, like to get a meeting together, and
> I always feel that I am being an inconvenience.
>
> (S30/T1/G7)

From an educational perspective, not having feedback left some students without information about their competence or performance.

5.4.2 Choosing who grades practice

Several students expressed the view that a different mentor might have affected their grade and that there was some element of choice in who graded them.

> I just wanted to make the point.... I just think that I come out of [the] tri-partite knowing that if I'd had a different mentor in there, I would have got a completely different mark (S19/T3/G5).
>
> So have I, and in some ways, you can choose your mentor to get a better mark (S22/T2/G5).

Despite what the students said, the practice grades were similarly high regardless of who assessed the student. Therefore, the impression that different mentors would award completely different grades was mistaken. S19 was articulate but quietly reserved in practice, with an earlier degree, would probably have been awarded a high practice grade by any mentor as all mentors seemed to respond well to her. However, for under-performing students, it may have been the difference between pass and refer grades.

The element of choice was discussed further by this 78-week student.

> It's difficult when you take one mentor, and obviously, we get to choose so we'll pick the one who's most likely to give us obviously, the best mark, in all honesty, but it also tended to be the one who you were on placement with at that time, so that obviously … cause if you said, 'Oh do you remember me I was out with you in March', you know will you come and sign this bit of paper … You could choose whomever you want, but obviously, you've been working with them over the last three or four weeks it was then in your interest to have them there.
>
> (S14/T2/G4S)

The students had contrasting views on choice. Some three-year students who knew their mentors for longer by being in practice more may have understood the system and known how to negotiate a different, preferred, mentor. Whereas, this 78-week student had a more pragmatic view of who was best placed to grade her practice.

To follow up on the student's points, a further analysis of the PADs was undertaken to see where the practice grades were undertaken and whether there was a deviation from the expected last placement of that year. Three 78-week students (Sf/T1, Sg/T1 and Sh/T1) had CDS mentors grade their final placement instead of mentors where they last worked. Some of these anomalies might be explained by the allocation plan. Grading should occur in a dedicated assessment week; however, mentors might be unavailable due to leave or days off in that specific week. Alternatively, there may have been an element of student choice.

As qualified nurses, it could be hypothesised most would feel comfortable in hospital settings and prefer hospital mentors, despite that none had MLBU mentors when four of the seven students were allocated there for their final placement. An interpretation of this is that students only have one placement on MBLU so prefer to go back to a mentor they are more familiar with, which in the last year was CDS where they had three placements. Most of these students' placements were in the hospital 35 (CDS, ward and MLBU) compared to 14 on the community. Therefore, the ten graded hospital placements compared to four community placements largely reflected their allocated placements.

Of the 19 students' PADs examined in the three-year cohort, all bar one had their practice graded in the community setting. Five students had their community mentor grade their practice on each summative occasion; they had not always worked most recently with their community mentor prior to the grading process. There were 14 end-of-year placements in the community, yet 30 graded assessments taken there. There should have been 27 CDS mentor assessments, but there were only 21 and four MLBU assessments but only two. This could be interpreted as students avoiding having their practice graded in the hospital environment when they should have done.

A potential reason for this is that more three-year students preferred the community; they developed better relationships with their community mentors and actively chose these mentors to grade their practice. Given that they had more timely feedback from these placements, this is not necessarily surprising. However, it does not reflect all their midwifery skills. While there may have been some choice, it is likely the students would have been awarded a high practice grade whomever they had, though knowing the mentor better might have helped increase their final grades. However, this could be considered a manipulation of the grading process bought about by having only one summative grade per year long practice module at Sanderling University Other universities also had this model with one grade per year, although there was also variation in the frequency of graded episodes across the UK (Fisher, et al. 2017).

5.5 Competence and performance models of assessment

This chapter has analysed the student's practice grades, showing that most students receive a first for practice. This was despite Sanderling University having three grading tools during the case study. While the second version of the tool increased the student's grades, they all enabled most students to be awarded a first. There was a great deal of discussion about the terminology and banding of first-class grades on the final iteration. This version meant some students' grades were slightly lower, but the majority were still awarded firsts.

Bernstein (1990) compares competence and performance models. He says that performance can be graded according to how well a student meets the criteria. While some mentors understood the assessment criteria, others apparently needed this interpreted, sometimes by the student. The opportunity for students to influence the grading process when they explained grading to their mentors was noted by some students. Hence, it could be argued that the criteria are not explicit enough, and they need to be according to Bernstein for a graded performance. A graded performance should stratify students; however, in this research, there was minimal stratification of grades as the majority were clustered at the top of the scale, as is the case with other research (Scanlan and Care, 2004; Seldomridge and Walsh, 2006; Walsh and Seldomridge, 2005; Edwards, 2012).

In a performance model, the grade awarded is not transferrable to another area, so the grade has no value in the next area of practice (Bernstein, 2000). The students thought they should be assessed in each area of practice too, since their performance in the community did not relate to their practice in the hospital. Competence assessment, alternatively, crosses the boundaries. My reading of the grades is that the mentor is authorising the student as progressing as expected rather than grading their practice, so the assessment is a competence model rather than a performance model.

The process of self-assessing their own performance, the confidence to do this, and the sense of self-disclosure students experienced differed with each iteration of the grading tool. Students engaged impression management strategies so they were not considered over- or under-confident, knowing this might affect their grade. The pedagogic discourse, which includes the regulative rule, was discussed to show that a lack of confidence in an area of practice was detrimental to the evaluation of the students' performance (Bernstein, 1990). Therefore, students were right to worry about the impression's mentors formed of them in practice.

Mentors too had to appear confident in the grading process for students to feel reassured by their assessment. Students tended to self-assess their performance slightly lower than their mentors. Mentor's tended to raise the student's grades. This may increase students' confidence in practice. Generally, students closer to qualification were awarded higher grades for practice.

The three-year students often felt more confident in the community environment. Here, the timeliness of feedback was better than in the hospital. The relationship with the community mentor, which was often closer than with hospital staff, may have helped this. It may have also affected where students' final assessments were undertaken. Most three-year students had their practice graded by their community mentor. Whereas, the 78-week students tended to have more hospital placements graded. This pattern did not always match the allocated final placement; therefore, one could argue that some students seemed to have the authority to choose who graded their practice. The practice grade was a culmination of one year's placements, so the students could have argued that the grade encompassed the majority of their work, if not all of it.

The social interactions between students and mentors clearly affected the grading practices. The implication of grading as a social process is that it enables some students to negotiate who grades their practice and others unable to shows inequality in the educational system. It is the effect of the pedagogic device, in who gets access to what and how.

When students received a lower practice grade this often affected their self-esteem and possibly their commitment to the profession. Some lower grades were due to explicit unwelcome interference from the lecturer. The authority of the lecturer seemed to assert more power than the mentor in practice despite the mentor knowing the student's capabilities. The students who were referred in practice will be considered in more detail in the following chapter.

Bibliography

Bernstein, B., (1990). *Class, Codes and Control Volume VI The Structuring of Pedagogic Discourse*. London: Routledge Taylor and Francis Group.

Bernstein, B., (2000). *Pedagogy, Symbolic Control and Identity Theory, Research, Critique*. 2nd ed. Oxford: s.n.

Briscoe, G. W., Carlson, D. L., Arcand, L. A., Levine, R E. & Cohen, M. J. (2006). Clinical grading in psychiatric clerkships. *Academic Psychiatry*, 30(2), pp. 104–109.

Chenery-Morris, S., (2011). Evaluating grading in practice away day-University Campus Suffolk. *MIDIRS*, 21(1), pp. 22–24.

Edwards, A., (2012). Grading practice: An evaluation one year on. *Nurse Education Today*, 32(6), pp. 627–629.

Goffman, E., (1959). *Presentation of Self in Everyday Life*. New York: Doubleday Anchor.

Gray, M. & Donaldson, J., (2009a). *Exploring Issues in the Use of Grading in Practice; Literature Review Final Report Volume 1*. Edinburgh: Edinburgh Napier University.

Gray, M. & Donaldson, J., (2009b). *Exploring Issues in the Use of Grading in Practice; Literature Review Final Report Volume 2*. Edinburgh: Edinburgh Napier University.

Heaslip, V. & Scammell, J. M., (2012). Failing underperforming students: The role of grading in practice assessment. *Nurse Education in Practice*, 12(2), pp. 95–100.

Hiller, K. M., Waterbrook, A. & Waters, K., (2016). Timing of emergency medicine student evaluation does not affect scoring. *Journal of Emergency Medicine*, 50(2), pp. 302–307.

Hivid Jacobson, M. & Kristiansen, S., (2015). *The Social Thought of Erving Goffman*. London: SAGE Ltd.

Hunt, L., McGee, P., Gutteridge, R. & Hughes, M., (2012). Assessment of student nurses in practice: A comparison of theoretical and practical assessment results in England. *Nurse Education in Practice*, 32(4), pp. 351–355.

Lawson, L., Jung, J. & Hiller, K., (2016). Clinical assessment of medical students in emergency medicine clerkships: A survey of current practice. *Journal of Emergency Medicine*, 51(6), pp. 705–711.

Murphy, S., Dalton, M. & Dawes, D., (2014). Assessing physical therapy students' performance during clinical practice. *Physiotherapy Canada*, 66(2), pp. 169–176.

NMC, (2009). *Standards for Pre-Registration Midwifery Education*. London: Nursing and Midwifery Council.

Plakht, Y., Shiyovich, A., Nusbaum, L. & Raizer, H., (2013). The association of positive and negative feedback with clinical performance, self-evaluation and practice contribution of nursing students. *Nurse Education Today*,33(10), pp. 1264–1268.

Roden, P., (2016). Do occupational therapy graduates benefit from grade inflation on practice placements?. *British Journal of Occupational Therapy*, 77(3), pp. 134–138.

Scammell, J., Halliwell, D. & Partlow, C., (2007). *Assessment of Practice in Pre-Registration Undergraduate Nursing Programmes: An Evaluation of a Tool to Grade Student Performance in Practice*. Bournemouth: Bournemouth University.

Scanlan, J. M. & Care, W. D., (2004). Grade inflation: Should we be concerned? *Journal of Nursing Education*, 43(10), pp. 475–478.

Seldomridge, L. A. & Walsh, C. M., (2006). Evaluating student performance in undergraduate preceptorships. *Journal of Nursing Education*, 45(5), pp. 169–176.

Walsh, C. M. & Seldomridge, L. A., (2005). Clinical grades: Upward bound. *Journal of Nursing Education*, 44(4), pp. 162–168.

Wolff, R. P., (2007). A discourse on grading. In: R. Curren, ed. *Journal of Philosophy of Education*. Oxford: Blackwell Publishing Ltd, pp. 489–464.

6 Students with practice referrals or concerns

This chapter examines in detail students who were referred in practice and those who had concerns about their practice documented. The study included ten student cases who were referred in practice. Seven students were on the three-year programme and three on the 78-week programme. Students who were referred were given a further placement of at least four weeks, with the same or different mentor, for their practice to be reassessed. After the second practice opportunity, two students, one from each programme, were failed and withdrawn due to practice failure. The other eight students passed practice and qualified as midwives. When students were failed and withdrawn, they usually kept their PADs, so the qualitative evidence from this data source was not available for the case study. However, evidence from five students' PADs, who later passed, have been analysed.

In addition, evidence to support this chapter is derived from an analysis of 12 students' action plans, including one of the students who was failed and withdrawn. Action plans were generated when a mentor saw a student was under-performing during a placement, prior to the summative assessment of their practice. The mentor would usually contact a lecturer and arrange a meeting with the student and lecturer to discuss the student's progress and concerns about their practice. An action plan would be written after the meeting, detailing the underperformance or concern(s). This was to ensure the student, mentor, and lecturer had an agreed measure of performance success against which to evaluate the student's progress.

Progress would be formally reviewed, often on a fortnightly basis, by the student, mentor, and lecturer, and the action plan updated. When a student proved they had met the expected performance on the action plan, the skill deficits were 'signed off' as completed, and the student passed the placement. However, it was possible for a student on an action plan to have new issues raised and documented. All the issues had to be resolved for the student to pass. If the student did not meet the expectations, they were referred in practice, and a further placement was organised to increase the student's exposure to midwifery practice prior to reassessment. Some of the students who had action plans developed withdrew from the course before the end of their practice placement. However, the majority who persevered passed and qualified as midwives.

The literature to support this chapter is derived mainly from nursing (Duffy, 2004; Scanlan and Chernomas, 2016; Lewallen and DeBrew, 2012; Killam et al.,

2011), or nursing education and social work (Luhanga et al., 2014). There is a paucity of research on under-performing midwifery students or reasons for practice failure. Therefore, this chapter presents new knowledge. However, there are marked similarities between reasons students were referred in other professional programmes and midwifery students' practice issues. These will be discussed after the empirical evidence.

6.1 Student case 1: Multiple practice concerns, failed and withdrawn

Table 6.1 illustrates the grades and areas where concerns were raised for S22/T2/G5's practice. She was referred (R) in practice at the end of the second and third year. After reassessment, she passed her second year with a capped practice grade (3–). However, she was failed and withdrawn from the programme prior to qualification. While her PAD was not available for analysis, action plans were generated by mentors in almost every area of midwifery practice (Community, CDS in both years and MLBU), as Table 6.1 denotes. S22/T2/G6's multiple action plans detailed examples of her difficulty in decision-making and a lack of confidence. For instance, in the community, she was unsure of what care to offer women during antenatal appointments at different gestations. Her lack of confidence meant she did not always finish consultations with women, and she looked to the mentor to complete the appointment. This was not considered an acceptable performance by her mentor, and so an action plan was developed, so she knew what she had to achieve on reassessment.

She experienced ill health and had several weeks of sick leave. Three months prior to her expected qualification date a mentor, on MLBU, on her second practice attempt said she was not safe to practice. S22/T2/G6 had forgotten to listen to the fetal heart when admitting a woman in labour, and had not expected birth despite changes in the woman's behaviour. The mentor judged the student's performance as unsafe to practice. Consequently, she was failed and withdrawn from the course.

Table 6.1 Student 1 with multiple practice concerns

Student	Second-year placements where concerns raised	Practice grade	Final-year placements where concerns raised	Practice grade
S22/T2/G5	Community/CDS	R/3–	CDS/MLBU	R/R withdrawn

6.2 Students who subsequently passed practice

Table 6.2 differs from Table 6.1 as each of the five students represented were only referred on their final placement. However, S32/T1/G7 had concerns raised about her performance on CDS in her second and third year, and Se/T3 was noted to

Table 6.2 Students who qualified despite referring practice

Student	First six months/second-year placement where concern raised	Practice grade	Final-year placement(s) where concern(s) raised	Practice grade
Se/T3	No concerns	2:2+	CDS, Ward	R/3–
S31/T3/G7	No concerns	DM/2:2–	Community	R/3–
S32/T1/G7	CDS	DM/2:2–	CDS	R/3–
Sm/T3	No concerns	1–	CDS	R/3–
Sn/T1	No concerns	DM/2:1+	CDS	R/3–

be under-performing in two areas in her final year. Three students needed more time to complete their second year (depicted in the Defer Mitigation (DM)). This was due to a lack of opportunity to demonstrate skills rather than issues with their practice. However, on further analysis it may have been a lack of mentor confidence to refer the students' practice and more time requested instead. This will be explored.

Given that most students received a first or 2:1 grade for practice, the three 2:2 grades are suggestive of under-performing students, and the analysis of their PADs and action plans is necessary to explore their issues. During this analysis, it was noted that Sn/T1 had several communication and confidence issues documented in her PAD, which should have been reflected in her practice grade. Her practice grade of 2:1+ masks these concerns.

6.2.1 Communication concerns and a lack of confidence

Three students, Sn/T1, S32/T1/G7, on the three-year programme, and Se/T3, a 78-week student, had concerns with communication skills and confidence raised. How these manifested and affected their performance was individual.

Student case 2

Continuity of mentorship was documented as problematic for Se/T3. The mentor, at the mid-point meeting, on the student's first placement recorded:

> [Student's name] is putting herself under a lot of pressure to learn everything all at once and to perform to a very high level. This at times could make [name] vulnerable and compromise her ability to learn as 'a student'.'
>
> (Se/T3 PAD)

The use of inverted commas and meaning behind the mentor's comments are ambiguous; I interpreted them to symbolise an intense student, and the mentor was trying to control the amount of learning the student was exposed to.

However, seen in the context of the final placement review their meaning can be understood to signify an issue with different forms of communication.

> [Student's name] needs to be less afraid of asking questions to enhance her learning as a student. She needs support with writing midwifery documentation in a concise and accurate way, as English is not her first language. As previously discussed, [student's name] is putting herself under immense pressure to perform at a very high level instead of allowing herself to take a step back to listen and learn and enjoy being a student midwife.
>
> (Se/T3 PAD)

The inability to ask questions may have been a reaction to the mid-point interview where the student was informed she was putting herself under too much pressure, and the student stopped showing her interest in every detail. As stated in Chapter 4, students respond to interactions with mentors to meet their mentors' expectations. Several of the communication issues noted in the 78-week students' PADs referred to English as their second language. The communication manner, thick accent, or speed of translation was the cause of the problem rather than an inability to communicate in English. For Se/T3, it was documenting in English. The limitations in Se/T3's practice appear to be reflected in the first practice grade (2:2+).

No further issues were documented in Se/T3's PAD until three months before she was due to qualify. The action plan generated by her CDS mentor detailed a lack of assertiveness that meant Se/T3 had not achieved all her practice competencies, and she needed 23 further births in her remaining two weeks. To enable the student time to achieve her births and competencies, her placement was extended.

On her final ward placement, the mentor recognised Se/T3 needed substantial supervision and a further action plan and placement time was needed. She was unable to prioritise care, lacked induction of labour and pelvic floor knowledge, and had many skills left to be completed. This meant her placement was extended beyond the original course plan. Her practice was referred, and on reassessment a capped grade of 40% was awarded. The decision to refer Se/T3's practice was administrative rather than an individual midwife's authority. There were no extenuating circumstances; the student had not met the programme outcomes within the course timeframe due to limitations in her knowledge and skills.

Student case 3

S32/T1/G7 had an action plan generated in the second and third years due to her inability to communicate appropriately on CDS; she was too quiet. This was considered a barrier to her handing over care, relating to other professionals, and supplying information and informed choice to women. She needed extra time to complete her second- and third-year competencies and considerable ongoing support, which was documented on her third-year action plan. Her practice grades were low, which is congruous with limited communication skills. In her final placement on CDS she was unable to show all the skills required of her by the course completion date and was referred in practice because she had no extenuating circumstances to mitigate for her lack of skills. With extra time and support she later passed.

During the group discussion, she barely contributed, but this was a particularly talkative group which included several vocal students wanting to share their experiences. Interestingly, several of the students in Group 7 had issues in practice. They may have chosen to take part in the group interview together as they had a shared identity; one of not quite meeting their mentors' expectations or as a student struggling in practice. When she did contribute, she disclosed she was stressed by the practice environment:

> I went into the community first, and I'm kind of glad I did that as it was a lot less manic and stressful than working in the hospital. And it is more one-to-one care than looking after a whole bay of people.
>
> (S32/T1/G7)

S32/T1/G7 used strong words to describe her hospital experience. The term stressful was used by several other students but in relation to getting their assessments completed, not the environment itself. She also said she had emotional support from one of her mentors and that they became friends (presented in Chapter 4). This is likely to have contributed to her eventual success.

Student case 4

On her first community placement, Sn/T1's mentor documented:

> Increase awareness of own opinions and how those may conflict with those of clients- practice acceptance.
>
> (Sn/T1's PAD)

The mentor's comments imply the student was outspoken, and her advice suggested that the student should be more accepting of women's choices. Her opinions caused relationship problems on her next placement as the ward mentor documented:

> [Students name] is beginning to relax and bring down the barriers which come across as over-confidence. This is improving relationships and abilities to teach/ learn.
>
> (Sn/T1's PAD)

Within the first five months on the course the student had been named as overconfident and outspoken by two separate mentors. However, this was not reflected in her practice grade (2:1+).

During her final year, concerns about Sn/T1's over-confidence in the hospital setting were raised again. A meeting was convened with the student, mentor, and lecturer to discuss the issue. Sn/T1, however, expressed a lack of confidence within the hospital and due to the different interpretations of her practice, no formal action plan was developed. Following this meeting, Sn/T1 had frequent sickness from practice and rarely worked a full week in the hospital setting.

When Sn/T1 met with her CDS mentor for her final review, she still had outstanding practice hours and births to complete. The student requested an extension of her training due to a lack of opportunity of births and sickness. However, the mentor said she was under pressure from senior CDS midwives to refer the student's practice. Her practice was evaluated to lack recognition of deviations from the normal and initiation of appropriate care plans. She had also not adhered to the doctor's plan of care for the woman she attended. Accordingly, she was considered unsafe to practice. The concerns had not been previously expressed to the student, so she was unaware she would be referred.

During the reassessed placement, Sn/T1 maximised her chance of success by negotiating to work with one particular midwife. She also devised a daily record sheet that she asked the mentor to complete. Upon reassessment, she presented the daily records as evidence that she was safe to practice.

6.2.2 Mentor authority in relationships with students

These three students, and S22/T2/G6, had similar issues raised about their characteristics (confidence) and aspects of care (communication skills, recognising deviations); however, unlike S22, these students qualified. The differences between the cases can be explored with respect to mentor authority and the number of times concerns were formally raised and documented. S22/T2/G6 had four separate mentors document her limitations in practice and initiate action plans. Similarly, Se/T3 and S32/T1/G7 had two action plans generated by mentors. However, S22/T2/G6's final mentor actively decided to terminate her training as she had had sufficient opportunities to demonstrate effective midwifery care and still the student was unable to. The mentors for Se/T3 and S32/T1/G7 recognised the students' practice limitations, documented these, and awarded grades consistent with the students' performance, but the decision to refer both students was administrative. They had not completed their practice competencies in the expected time and had therefore not initially passed.

Conversely, Sn/T1's initial practice grade masked any concerns previously documented in her PAD. This is evidence of a disparity between the qualitative and quantitative evaluation of this student's practice. She did not have an action plan generated until she was referred in practice on her final placement, despite several mentor's concerns. Instead of a lack of confidence, she was perceived to be overconfident. It was perhaps this characteristic that prevented mentors from generating an action plan sooner. Section 1.4 discussed research that showed assessors reluctance to give candid feedback to students, especially dealing with unhappy or angry students (Briscoe et al., 2006; Fazio et al., 2013). The student's authority may have inhibited mentors from developing a formal action plan. Mentors documented some of their practice concerns but did not act on these.

Sn/T1 expected to be granted an extension for her practice and enabled extra time. However, pressure from senior midwives meant her mentor was advised to refer Sn/T1's practice instead. The mentor had the authority to ignore the senior midwives; however, she accepted their concerns, perhaps because there would have been consequences for her relationships with her colleagues if she had not listened. The mentor explained the reasons for the referral to Sn/T1 and in doing so distanced herself from the decision. In this way, she used the authority of others more senior to her for the assessment outcome.

6.2.3 Lack of knowledge and inappropriate attitude

The other two students, S31/T3/G7 and Sm/T3, showed a lack of knowledge at the end of their course. This was combined with inappropriate assertiveness or attitudinal problems.

Student case 5

Sm/T3 had an action plan developed after a lack of knowledge was demonstrated on the third stage of labour. The student said she had been taught incorrectly and did not accept responsibility for this deficit in knowledge. This generated 'talk' of her seemly unprofessional attitude for several months prior to this incident, and the mentor who was allocated to support her was under pressure from her peers to fail the student (email communication between the mentor and lecturers). Five key issues were noted. She was considered unable to prioritise care and keep up with the documentation, demonstrate proficiency with all aspects of the midwife's role, show a good understanding of an obstetric emergency, knowledge of neonatal resuscitation, or blood results. It was also recorded that she did not prove a willingness to admit her strengths and weaknesses.

Looking through the extensive documentation from Sm/T3s action plans, the essence of the problem was never really articulated. An excerpt from one of the many mentor emails, quoted with consent, explains the problem:

> In general, I am concerned that [student's name] attitude has not changed at all. She comes across as a very negative person at times and seems to be very happy complaining about people whether they are midwives or university lecturers! At this juncture, I am not happy to sign her off and would not want my name and status as a midwife to be associated with her entry onto the professional register. As you can appreciate, this whole experience has been fairly stressful for me as I am not a naturally negative person and prefer to give people the benefit of the doubt and see the best in them. However, I feel that I am unable to do this for [student's name] as a result of her behaviour and because of the list of concerns I have about her.

The mentor went on to list how many skills Sm/T3 had left to achieve and how indifferent the student appeared by these. Until five months before qualification there had been no issues at all recorded with this student. Nevertheless, once one was recorded a catalogue of other issues then seemed to appear, all of which masked the real problem; that of her attitude. Had the attitudinal problem been documented, the criteria for success would have been visible to the student, and she would have had a greater opportunity to develop more professional behaviours.

Sm/T3 and her mentor needed substantial support from the university lecturers for the reassessed CDS placement. Pressure on the mentor to fail the student continued from other staff on CDS, including the ward manager. On reassessment, the mentor documented: 'I feel the student has proved herself as [a] safe and competent practitioner' (Sm/T3 PAD). The change from positional status noted in the mentor's email to personal verification of the student's practice is clear. The student and mentor worked for several months together and during this time, even with a student who has limitations, the relationship classification and framing strength altered. Despite ongoing concerns about Sm/T3's manner, it became harder for Sm/T3's mentor to fail the student as she accomplished all her action plan targets.

Student case 6

By contrast, S31/T3/G7, was not assertive enough in getting her PAD and skills signed; however, she experienced poor continuity of mentorship on several placements, and this may have affected her ability to complete her documentation. All three of her first-year placements were evaluated late, with one four months after the placement had finished. A minor concern was documented in the first year: the student needed to be more assertive in initiating conversations with women. Her second-year grade (2:2) suggested there were areas for practice development; however, no action plan was developed. The lack of timely feedback and inconsistent mentorship may have decreased S31/T3/G7's knowledge and opportunities to acquire and demonstrate practice knowledge.

In her final year community placement, S31/T3/G7 asked me to attend her mid-point interview to help keep her 'on track'. I soon realised she wanted me to help manage her community mentor. With three months until she was due to qualify, there were 100 competencies unsigned, mostly related to community skills and drug administration. The community mentor had concerns about S31's lack of knowledge relating to fetal screening and dietary advice and the ability to offer information to women. These forms of communication with women are usually developed in the first year, as presented in Chapter 3, so the mentor was right to express concern. She also said that the student's attitude was too casual, although this was not stated on the action plan. Due to these apprehensions, the mentor was reluctant to sign any of S31's skills. The placement was extended, but the student was still unable to show all the skills required of her, so she was referred. Upon reassessment, with a different mentor, she passed.

S31/T3/G7 was frustrated that her mentor refused to sign any skills in her PAD and discussed this at each action plan review with examples and reflections from cases that she thought proved her ability to provide care. The mentor, probably due to the presence of a lecturer at the review meetings, reluctantly signed one or two skills on each visit. This was a symbolic act as there were still too many unsigned skills for the student to qualify. The decision to change the student to another mentor was initiated by the community mentor who articulated work pressures as a rationale for the change. It may have been a strategy to avoid failing the student. The student agreed, and the new mentor seemed more confident in the student's ability. The mentor offered S31/T3/G7 more opportunities to show her skills, and therefore she qualified.

6.2.4 The regulative discourse

The development of an action plan should mean the limitations in these students' practice were made more explicit and visible to the student, mentor, and lecturer. For many students, their lack of knowledge or documentation skills were relatively easy to improve. However, action plans reduced the concerns into examples of what the student needs to demonstrate to succeed; they were reductive. A successful student performance in practice is greater than the examples on the action plan, especially when the problem was not *what* but *how* care was delivered. Several of the students had concerns about how care was delivered; this was in relation to how quiet, assertive, or confident they were. It was these issues, the manner of the student which were not always expressed.

When students achieved all the NMC competencies and completed the action plan points, they should pass practice. However, both the mentors for S31/T3 and Sm/T3 expressed concerns that neither the action plans nor the NMC Essential Skills Clusters, the criteria by which the students were judged, were adequate for assessing the students' total performance.

Bernstein (1990) discusses the skills and values of the education system in pedagogic discourses. He explains that the division of skills and values is a conspiracy as there is, in his theory, only one discourse. The instructional discourse that transmits the necessary skills is always embedded in the regulative discourse, which is the values. The way the students undertook midwifery practice, whether they were too assertive or too casual in their approaches, affected the evaluation of their performance. Behind Bernstein's theory is Durkheim's analysis of the medieval university in the West (Moore, 2013): the division between the Trivium and Quadrivium or mechanical and organic solidarity, which in turn signify the inner and outer or sacred and profane. How the students delivered midwifery care was not acceptable as the inner student values affected the care delivered; the inner was present in the outer. The co-existence of the sacred and profane within the same individual and as part of their identity is the essence of the pedagogic discourse.

Only one of the five student cases presented in this section continued to work at the Trust once qualified. The other four applied for and were appointed at

Trusts outside the local area. One interpretation I have of this is that students' identities were disrupted when their practice was referred, especially when this was related to who they were as people: to their inner self. Once qualified employment in another Trust enabled the registrant to recreate their identity in relation to other qualified midwives and they had greater chance to 'be themselves'.

6.3 Overview of other students' action plans

Table 6.3 depicts six other students who had an action plan generated. Three of the students withdrew from the course with an impending referral in practice in their third year (S27/T1/G6, S30/T1/G7, Sr/T2). Concerns had been documented about all three students in their second year, and each had considerable absence from practice due to illness during their course. The lack of practice knowledge could have been a result of fewer opportunities to learn midwifery due to absences. Conversely, the absences may have been a manifestation of the stress these students experienced when concerns were raised about their practice.

The students who withdrew had the following practice issues documented on their action plans: lack of professional language, anxiety affecting the ability to work on CDS, not able to prioritise the workload, a lack of confidence and possible avoiding behaviours. These issues can be attributed to the regulative discourse: the manner of the student was judged by mentors to be lacking some professional attribute. One of the students also disclosed ineffective mentoring (presented in Section 4.2) that could be interpreted as bullying. The ineffective mentoring/bullying affected her ability to acquire practice knowledge and probably contributed to her decision to withdraw from the course.

Table 6.3 Sample of other students whose practice warranted an action plan

Student	First six months/second-year placement where concern raised	Practice grade	Final placement(s) where concern(s) raised	Practice grade
Sd/T2	No concerns	1–	CDS	1=
Sp/T3	Ward	2:1+	CDS, Ward	1–
S27/T1/G6	CDS	2:2+	CDS, ward, community	withdrew
S29/T2/G7	CDS	1–	No concerns	1+
S30/T1/G7	CDS	DM/2:1=	CDS	withdrew
Sr/T2	Ward	1=	ward	withdrew

6.3.1 *Student case 7*

Sp/T3 demonstrated unprofessional behaviours, including chewing gum at work, difficulties with punctuality, not always asking for permission to enter a private discussion or procedure, and not always upholding the uniform policy (wearing fabric instead of leather or plastic shoes). One incident where she did not report changes in a CTG quickly enough was also documented. Sp/T3 had multiple practice issues documented in her PAD by many mentors and three action plans developed. The mentor on CDS documented:

> Following discussions with co-mentors there is a unanimous feeling that her focus on CDS has been on achieving normal births and we all feel that the student would benefit from returning to this placement without the pressure to obtain births.

> (Sp/T3 PAD)

The collective mentor voice legitimised the decision for reassessment; however, it also shows how individual mentors seem reluctant to use their authority to fail students' practice.

Three points are made about this case, Sp/T3 was a nurse prior to her status as a midwifery student. This may have afforded her some authority or ability to negotiate with mentors' decisions. Therefore, the collective approach was taken. Similarly, as a nurse, she should have been familiar with the ward setting, but she still had two action plans developed there. While the work is different between nursing and midwifery, the routine and principles of professionalism are similar. It was the latter that were documented as problems for Sp/T3. Lastly, the framing of the need for a reassessed placement on CDS masks the authority of the mentor. Foregrounding the benefit for the student rather than limitations in their performance. This was seen in several students' PADs.

6.3.2 Summary of student cases

To summarise this section, reasons midwifery students were considered underperforming in practice included poor communication skills, a lack of confidence, inability to prioritise care, a lack of knowledge, lack of insight into behaviour, and poor professional behaviour. Concerns about the affective domain, communication, confidence, and professionalism, were most common. These can be understood as the manner of the student not embodying the professional midwifery role.

Several students had concerns raised in successive years or placements. This was often stressful for the student and manifested in absence from practice. A few students withdrew from the programme with impending practice referrals. For those that were referred in practice, the majority passed on reassessment. Only two students in the case study were failed and withdrawn. Five students were failed on their final placement, not all had concerns raised previously, or the concerns had not been formalised. This was particularly traumatic for the students and the mentors.

In total (across Tables 6.1, 6.2 and 6.3) 14 of the 24 action plans were generated on CDS. This suggests that understanding what is necessary for this area of practice is more difficult than the other areas where fewer action plans were generated. As students tended to receive delayed feedback from their CDS mentors, as discussed in Chapter 5, this could contribute to their anxiety in this area and have a detrimental effect on their performance and understanding of the requirements. Therefore, the higher rates of referral in this area can be explained. However, the relationship between the student and mentor will also affect the assessment of the student's practice; therefore, it could be that the mentors on CDS were more willing to assert their authority as gatekeepers, or that their slightly distanced relationship from the students enabled this.

6.4 Literature on student practice issues and referrals

There is evidence of characteristics of unsuccessful or failing nursing students in the literature (Lewallen and DeBrew, 2012; Killam et al., 2011; Scanlan and Chernomas, 2016; Duffy, 2004). An integrative literature review of 11 sources, albeit only six research studies, found ineffective interpersonal interactions, knowledge and skill incompetence, and unprofessional image as characteristics of failing nursing students (Killam et al., 2011). These characteristics are supported and developed further by more recent empirical evidence (DeBrew and Lewallen, 2014; Scanlan and Chernomas, 2016).

Critical incidents were collected from 24 nurse educators to describe their decision-making about student evaluations of failing students (DeBrew and Lewallen, 2014). A total of 25 incidents were described, including 10 students who passed and 15 who failed practice (DeBrew and Lewallen, 2014). The most common reason was poor communication skills. This encompassed written and verbal communication with staff, patients, and faculty. Not making progress was the second most common reason. This was followed by unsafe medicine management and inability to prioritise patient care, unsafe practice, and heightened student anxiety were also documented (DeBrew and Lewallen, 2014). The label unsafe to practice was explored in greater detail by Scanlan and Chernomas (2016).

Scanlan and Chernomas (2016) undertook a retrospective study of Canadian nursing students' files (n=51) who failed clinical practice over a six-year time span. Ten students were failed and withdrawn, 15 students withdrew voluntarily, and 26 students completed the nursing programme. Qualitative data from 19 student files was also examined, with a mix of student outcomes. Their study is similar to mine, in that retrospective PAD data were analysed, and in the proportion of students who passed, voluntarily withdrew and were failed and withdrawn.

Student anxiety and lack of self-confidence were interpreted as characteristics that interfered with the student's ability to learn and be successful in practice (Scanlan and Chernomas, 2016). These alone, or in combination with more easily seen behaviours, such a student's organisation, time management skills, and initiative, contributed to the mentor's assessment. Two of the students who withdrew in my study, one voluntarily and one who was failed, exhibited significant anxiety and a lack of confidence in practice that contributed to them leaving the course which was shown in the action plans.

Aspects of student practice that were seen in the failing students included communication problems, such as the inability to interact with patients

(Scanlan and Chernomas, 2016). A combination of individual and contextual factors resulted in a label of unsafe to practice (Scanlan and Chernomas, 2016). The individual presentation of unsafe practice was idiosyncratic. Scanlan and Chernomas (2016) described the phrase 'how students are in practice', their self-awareness, confidence, initiative, and anxiety, as features of student performance that were more difficult to discern and name. Moreover, they were also more difficult for the mentor to communicate to the student and for some students to accept and correct. If these aspects were communicated, the student was likely to succeed (Scanlan and Chernomas, 2016). In my study, how students were in practice was discussed in relation to the regulative discourse (Bernstein, 1990). The manner of the student was important. Sm/T3 especially did not receive feedback on her self-awareness until the final placement, and this almost affected her ability to qualify.

The aspects of practice, time management, communication, and care were typically measured in the students' practice assessment documentation. While the internal features of 'how the students are in practice' were not always part of the assessment tool (Scanlan and Chernomas, 2016). To succeed, they asserted, students needed these indicators named. Sanderling University's grading tools (Appendices 6–8) include aspects of student performance such as professionalism, ability to express personal feelings, confidence, and empathy as well as motivation, yet according to Sm/T3's mentor the student's attitude was not formally assessed through the university or NMC documentation. Perhaps attitude needs to be more explicitly assessed. Similarly, most often the students who were referred had been awarded high grades for those elements of professionalism earlier in their course. Therefore, either their attitude was not considered problematic or mentors chose not to bring attention to these elements of the student.

The authors noted one incongruent case in their analysis: a student who said the relationship with the mentor was the source of the practice problem (Scanlan and Chernomas, 2016). On the next placement, the student succeeded. The same outcome happened in my study with S31/T3/G7. Scanlan and Chernomas (2016) suggested further research into the importance of the mentoring relationship to success in clinical practice. My work contributes to the professional conversation about pedagogic relationships in midwifery.

A multidisciplinary qualitative study in Canada of 33 nursing, education, and social work professionals explored the failure to fail phenomenon in professional programmes (Luhanga et al., 2014). The findings included how difficult the process of failing students is, what support is needed for the student and mentor and how the reputation of the professions depends on making effective judgements about under-performing students. A range of generic risk indicators were identified that contributed to failing students in the final year, which were not easy to remedy. Red flags included, but were not limited to, unenthusiastic attitude, repetitive lateness, a high level of anxiety, a lack of confidence, a lack of knowledge and skills, poor documentation, a lack of insight into their behaviour, and an absence of professional boundaries or poor professional behaviour (Luhanga et al., 2014). Each profession also had their own specific indicators.

The seminal grounded theory research by Duffy (2004) of 14 lecturers and 26 nursing mentors, led to the label 'failing to fail'. The participants fell into three categories, those who had no experience of failing students, those who had failed a student, and those who later passed a student who had concerns against them. Her research noted, like mine, that mentors often expressed concerns but did not always act upon these. This meant students would almost complete the programme before a mentor was willing to refer the student. Therefore, the theme of leaving it too late was found (Duffy, 2004).

Early identification of student issues and the development of action plans offer the student the maximum opportunity to develop their clinical skills (Duffy, 2004). However, more than a decade later, it seems that several of the student cases presented in this chapter should have had action plans developed earlier, but due to mentor leniency or lack of confidence or authority this did not happen. Failing a student requires confidence, experience, and preparation, and many students were able to 'do enough to pass' (Duffy, 2004). Again, it seems that some of the students in my study knew how to navigate the system to enable them to pass, without amending the behaviours that caused the concerns to be raised. Some mentors may also have preferred to give students the 'benefit of the doubt' (Duffy, 2004). When students made some progress, mentors were more likely to pass them.

One interesting finding often overlooked in Duffy's (2004) work is the association between how many students fail theory compared to practice. This has been discussed in this study in Section 1.3.1; however, it calls for some discussion again here as some of these students referred many of their theoretical assessments as well as practice. The importance of good underpinning theory for practice is essential for all professionals.

Most of the student cases in my study, presented above, showed similar individual characteristics that affected differing aspects of their practice. Communication skills were documented most often. However, the findings presented in Chapter 3 and 4, show that many students assumed they had the requisite communication skills because they did not recognise the specific context of midwifery communication. Additionally, students had little feedback on these important skills. Therefore, it is not perhaps surprising that several students were unable to develop this skill in their pedagogic relationships. Contrary to the nursing literature, none of the students in my study were failed and withdrawn due to their communication skills. S22 was withdrawn due to unsafe practice.

The need to identify concerns early, to articulate these to the student to enable them to reflect on the issue, and, if possible, improve their performance before formally documenting and involving others were all noted to be good practice (Luhanga et al., 2014; Duffy, 2004). However, in my study, it seems that concerns were documented and presumably shared with the student, but sometimes no further action was taken. This was particularly problematic for the students who were perceived to be too assertive or overconfident. Participants in Luhanga et al.'s (2014) study cited reasons for failure to fail under-performing students, including avoiding vocal students and the time and effort required in mentoring a failing student. This was supported by other literature from medicine presented in Section 1.4 (Briscoe et al., 2006; Fazio et al., 2013).

Both Sm/T3 and Sn/T1 would have benefitted from earlier action plans about their personal characteristics and the way these affected upon aspects of their care. Failing students on their last placement, without having the opportunity to reflect on the issues is unfair to students and traumatic for all parties (Luhanga et al., 2014; Duffy, 2004). Had these issues been articulated sooner, I question whether each of these students would have passed, because the refer decision was on their final placement, I think the mentors had no choice but to pass the students.

While Sn/T1 had received some feedback about her communication skills and over-confidence, the lack of an action plan meant she had less time to work on her areas of weakness. Blaming others, lack of insight and acceptance of responsibility for one's practice, and an inability to reflect on practice were also cited in nursing students practice failures (Scanlan and Chernomas, 2016). Both students deflected their practice issues to problems outside themselves. Both blamed others for their difficulties. However, both passed because they met the conditions of their action plans and completed all NMC competencies.

6.5 The pedagogic discourse

Bernstein's pedagogic discourse can be used here to beneficial effect to show changes in the instructional and regulative discourses with these student–mentor relationships. To recap, the regulative discourse is concerned with the social order and manner of the student–teacher relationship (Bernstein, 2000). The instructional discourse is about the pacing and sequencing of knowledge (ibid). The two discourses come together in evaluating student's performances, but the regulative discourse, according to Bernstein, is always dominant. In this study deficits in students' knowledge (derived from the instructional discourse) were noted, more often though the problem was with the student's manner that resulted in a lower grade or referral in practice (the regulative discourse).

Several themes reoccurred in the students' action plans and PADs: communication deficits, prioritising care, decision-making, confidence, and some limited midwifery knowledge. At the outset of this work, I had expected a lack of knowledge to feature more often. However, using Bernstein, I can conclude that knowledge is not highly valued in clinical practice. The emphasis was on *how* students performed rather than *what* they knew. This emphasis on legitimate student's performances relates to Bernstein's regulative discourse. When deficits were noted, they were more often about a student's manner or authority; for instance, S22/T2/G5 lacked confidence and S31/T3/G7 was not assertive enough, whereas Sn/T1 was overconfident, and Sm/T3 was too assertive. More often, these attributes led to the generation of an action plan and referral in practice.

For some students, the explicit deficit noted in their action plan was easy to rectify, but for others the issue remained invisible, and the criteria for success remained elusive. This was in part down to mentor authority, where some mentors did not like to record the actual concerns and hid the attitudinal issues within other explicit concerns. The hierarchy between the student and mentor was often masked in these situations with mentors collectively deciding a student needed reassessment in practice. Some mentors were more direct; they demonstrated they were in a hierarchical position compared to the student and wrote early criticisms of student's deficits, even if they were related to attitudes.

From the evidence presented, most students seemed to respond positively to action plans and demonstrated a legitimate performance; however, some students left the course when practice issues were raised. Students with multiple deficits were more likely to leave, perhaps feeling their effort was futile, while most students who persevered qualified.

Several students on action plans had a noticeable lack of continuity of mentorship documented in the PADs, especially in their first year (S31/T3/G7, Se/T3, S29/T2/G7, Sp/T3). This may have been detrimental to their learning. It was certainly detrimental to their sense of belonging in clinical practice and to establish and build a relationship with a mentor, as presented in Chapter 4. Some students may be less able to cope with multiple mentors, especially early in their education when learning the basics. When access to knowledge is limited by the lack of relationship with a mentor, some students may be more likely to refer than others. As a profession, we have a responsibility to ensure each student reaches their potential.

Mentors sometimes documented a lack of continuity of mentorship with students, and this was used to mitigate student underperformance and sometimes mentor legitimacy of assessment. However, if the student performance did not improve their issues were escalated to an action plan. When a student's performance was reviewed on an action plan, mentor consistency became more important. This was twofold, to offer the student maximum opportunity to succeed by learning and demonstrating one mentor's preferred 'way', but also for the mentor to see student progress. However, many mentors, such as those for S31/T3/G7 and Sm/T3, found this relationship extremely intense and some tried not to have to decide on a student's final placement (such as S31/T3/G7's community mentor).

When the university lecturer became involved in the implementation and review of under-performing students, the lack of student progress became more visible to other students and mentors working in the department. The meetings were undertaken in private, but the reason for the increased presence of the lecturer was often known. This had the potential to generate talk about 'the under-performing student'. Midwives may talk amongst themselves to support one another to verify their concerns or the opinion that the student now has the capability to pass the placement. While there is some 'talk' of all students, the students on action plans are much more heavily scrutinised. This has two effects, students who are performing at the expected level are left to get on with the work, and those that are under-performing might feel inhibited to do anything without permission of their mentor. Learning the 'rules' of their mentor became even more important.

Students who were awarded a first for practice should have produced a legitimate practice performance. However, some students who had concerns about their practice were still awarded a first. These students may have had a good relationship with their mentor or weak hierarchy between the student and mentor. Students who had a lack of relationship seemed to be marked down, such as S31/T3/G7 and Se/T3 who were awarded 2:2 yet not on action plans initially. It could be argued that the mentors of these students were intuitive and noted an emerging problem, a lack of assertiveness for each student. I would argue that some students are not able to be assertive due to their personality or culture and a lack of continuity of mentor further compounds this. Some students seemed to be marked down because they did not fit the mentor's expected behaviour. Therefore, the grades, interpreted from the documentary data, were not solely about practice but authority, identity, and relationships.

Bibliography

Bernstein, B., (1990). *Class, Codes and Control Volume VI The Structuring of Pedagogic Discourse*. London: Routledge Taylor and Francis Group.

Bernstein, B., (2000). *Pedagogy, Symbolic Control and Identity Theory, Research, Critique*. 2nd ed. Oxford: Rowman and Littlefield Publishing Group inc.

Briscoe, G. W., Carlson, D. L., Arcand, L. A., Levine, R. E. & Cohen, M. J. (2006). Clinical grading in psychiatric clerkships. *Academic Psychiatry*, 30(2), pp. 104–109.

DeBrew, J. K. and Lewallen, L. P., (2014). To Pass or to Fail? Understanding the factors considered by faculty in the clinical evaluation of nursing students. *Nurse Education Today*, 34, pp. 631–636.

Duffy, K., (2004). *A Grounded Theory Investigation of Factors Which Influence the Assessment of Students' Competence to Practice*. London: Nursing and Midwifery Council.

Fazio, S. B., Papp, K. K., Torre, D. M. & DeFer, T. M., (2013). Grade inflation in the internal medicine clerkship: A national survey. *Teaching and Learning in Medicine*, 25(1), pp. 71–76.

Killam, L. A., Luhanga, F. & Bakker, D., (2011). Characteristics of unsafe undergraduate nursing students in clinical practice: An integrative literature review. *Journal of Nursing Education*, 50(8), pp. 437–446.

Lewallen, L. P. & DeBrew, K. J., (2012). Successful and unsuccessful clinical nursing students. *Journal of Nursing Education*, 51(7), pp. 389–395.

Luhanga, F. L., Larocque, S., MacEwan, L., Gwekwerere, Y. N. & Danyluk, P., (2014). Exploring the issue of failure to fail in professional education programmes; a multidisciplinary study. *Journal of University Teaching and Learning Practice*, 11(2), pp. 1–24.

Moore, R., (2013). *Basil Bernstein The Thinker and the Field*. Abingdon: Routledge.

NMC, (2009). *Standards for Pre-Registration Midwifery Education*. London: Nursing and Midwifery Council.

Scanlan, J. M. & Chernomas, W. M., (2016). Failing clinical practice and the unsafe student: A new perspective. *International Journal of Education Scholarship*, 13(1), pp. 109–116.

7 Conclusions about midwifery practice knowledge, relationships, identity and authority

This concluding chapter is separated into four parts. Initially, Bernstein's pedagogic codes will be explored further to explain the significance of the pedagogic discourse and device through structural relations and interactional practices. Then the nature of midwifery knowledge will be explored to show whether practice knowledge can be elaborated and therefore graded. Recommendations for the future will be offered. The concluding section will reflect on the study, its strengths and limitations as a sole-authored case study, and my research journey to draw the themes of relationships, identity, and authority together. This will include the relationship between the means I used to gain knowledge of others and the knowledge itself. To begin a review of the research questions.

1. What counts as valid midwifery practice knowledge?
2. What meaning do students and mentors attribute to the practice grade?
3. Is there a difference, real or perceived, between the quantitative grades awarded and qualitative feedback given to students?
4. What else is happening in the interactions between students and mentors that may be affecting the relationship or grade?

The concepts of classification (structural relations) and framing (interactional practices) presented in the earlier chapters were needed to explore grading practices because pedagogic codes regulate access to knowledge for diverse types of learners in separate ways. This means student practice grades should have been stratified; however, they tended to be similarly high. The grades could not be explored independently of the knowledge necessary for midwifery practice or teaching and learning; therefore, each of these aspects was covered in separate chapters.

Chapter 3 explored the first research question. Aspects of the official knowledge principally determined by the NMC (2009) were either upheld or minimalised locally in the practice settings. Communication and interpersonal skills were not valued as much by students as specific clinical skills because the students thought they already had these affective skills. This was largely substantiated by the mentors in feedback in students' PAD. Students wanted access to, and to be able to practise clinical skills; they saw these as specialised knowledge and essential to the role of the midwife. By contrast, using evidence to inform practice was considered students' work; therefore, it was not highly valued in practice despite the professional responsibility to offer evidence-based care.

What counted as valid midwifery practice knowledge depended upon the classification between agents, contexts, and practices. Students thought clinical skills counted, especially in the hospital environment. Whereas pregnant women valued the relationship with their midwife and communication skills. Due to the weak classification of affective domain skills, as students progressed through their course, they tended to value the more technical aspects of midwifery. This has implications for midwives' identities and will be discussed further. Similarly, when mentors encouraged students to develop into autonomous practitioners, they were foregrounding the student as a knower rather than reinforcing the underpinning knowledge and evidence for midwifery practice. This will be discussed further in section 7.3.2.

Chapter 4 considered the pedagogic relationship between a mentor and student in clinical practice. It answered the fourth research question. Differences were noted in students' access to learning or practice knowledge between distinct groups, such as those with previous formal nursing or informal care knowledge and those new to hospital environments. Interactions in practice were affected by the three rules of the pedagogic discourse. Bernstein (2000) defined the three rules in terms of hierarchy, sequencing and criteria. As one cannot teach someone else something they already know, the pedagogic relationship always entails a disparity between transmitters and acquirers in relation to the presence or absence of knowledge/practice/skills. A range of pedagogic relationships were presented with differences in the presence and absence of knowledge and from least to most visible control or hierarchy between mentors and students.

In relation to sequencing, explicit mentor control or strong framing reduced the students' ability to select and access practice knowledge. However, some students could alter the relationship between the mentor and themselves to reduce the hierarchy, which enabled greater access to learning. Not all students had this authority. The terms visible and invisible pedagogy were offered to show differences in mentor–student hierarchy, pacing, selection, and skill acquisition. Students usually preferred weak hierarchical structures between them and their mentor; this afforded more student-led learning and control. Some students understood this invisible pedagogy; others needed more explanation from their mentor to access midwifery knowledge. However, not all midwives explained, and some students were unable to ask for more detail.

Positive and negative mentor framing styles led to labels such as guiding or controlling. Bernstein calls this the regulative discourse and this is always dominant. It is *how* practice knowledge was transmitted. The other discourse, the instructional specialised midwifery knowledge, was discussed by students less often. This was *what* knowledge was transmitted. When students discussed how they acquired this specialised knowledge, it was usually in narratives which foregrounded strong or weak mentor control, rather than the knowledge itself. This too has implications for students' development of their midwifery identity and reinforces the knower stance.

Chapter 5 explored the evaluation of learning or criteria for assessment. It showed that most students were awarded a first for their practice grade and answered the second research question. High practice grades symbolised acceptance into the profession by mentors. This seemed to increase students' confidence in their practice and positive identity within the profession. Conversely, low practice grades, or a reduction in students' self-evaluated grades, had negative effects on students' personal and professional identity development.

My interpretation of the high practice grades is that most students produced a legitimate performance (or text) because they recognised the specific context. A text was anything that was evaluated; this included students' posture, attitude, or dress, as well as knowledge. Because the regulative discourse is dominant, it could be argued that the former features of the student, their personal qualities, were judged before the latter, knowledge. Using Bernsteinian theories, the high practice marks can be understood as similar competences between student midwives rather than stratified graded performances; usually mediated by weak classification between the student and mentor, especially at the end of the course. The students' personal qualities corresponded with the established orthodoxy, and therefore they were awarded high practice grades.

Chapter 6 explored the students whose practice was not considered first class. It answered research question 3. Some students with action plans, which symbolised areas of practice weakness, were still awarded high practice grades by their mentors. Individually mentors seemed to lack authority to refer students' practice or to award lower practice grades, or preferred not to. Thus, there was a disparity between some of the qualitative and quantitative feedback to students. The students often lacked theoretical midwifery knowledge, and this was detailed on their action plans. However, the students' ability to project a legitimate manner was usually the source of the concern. This issue was not always communicated to the student. When students were offered a second attempt to pass practice, often the mentor still awarded a high grade (although this was capped at the Assessment Board). This illustrates the difficulty in quantitatively and qualitatively assessing student midwives. Frequently students who were referred in practice left the profession either during their education or shortly after it. Those who chose to stay in midwifery often transferred to a different Trust where potentially their identity could be reconstructed.

This chapter will explore how the code affected different learners in each environment and the discourses this generated in practice. The practice environment was reported to be too busy to prioritise learning, the formal aspects of feedback prior to the graded assessment were not always adhered to, and relationships in midwifery practice were prioritised over knowledge. This meant that the differences between students were not discerned when practice was graded. This was corroborated by the practice grades as almost all students received a high mark. Therefore, my conclusion is that grading practice in its current form by mentors based on observation of students' practice is not robust or trustworthy.

As mentioned in Chapter 4, the NMC published new standards in 2018 that supersede the NMC (2008) *Standards for Learning and Assessment in Practice* (SLAiP). The new standards for student supervision and assessment (SSSA) separate the requirement to supervise students to learn from assessing students. The new terms 'practice supervisor' and 'practice assessor' will be used from 2020 for all midwifery curricula. To ensure this book reflects this change in terminology and remains current, I stop using the term mentor here. Preferring instead to use midwife. At times I include the new role nomenclature in brackets to illustrate how the discussion that ensues can be applied to the new practice assessment framework (NMC, 2018) and new midwifery proficiencies (NMC, 2019).

7.1 Bernstein's pedagogic code

Bernstein's (2000, p.187) pedagogic code will be explored further to articulate the concepts and their relationships to this project's focus: grading students' practice.

This is the code:

$$\frac{O_{E/R}}{+\text{-}C\ ie/+\text{-}F\ ie}$$

Figure 7.1 The pedagogic code.

O refers to orientation to elaborated (OE) or restricted (OR) meaning. An elaborate orientation has a universal meaning that is relatively independent of the context. In a restricted orientation, the meaning is particular and context-dependent. This is realised by classification (C), and framing (F), which can be strong (+) or weak (−), internal (i) or external (e). This formula explains the ability of the midwife (practice supervisor) to orientate meaning to the student in an elaborated or restricted way depending on the strength of classification and framing, between contexts (external) and within them (internal). Each time a code strength changes, from strong to weak, for instance, the orientation to meaning also changes.

Bernstein's pedagogic codes are used to discuss consequences for identity and identity change for both the learner and the midwife who embodies the role of either practice supervisor or practice assessor. A pedagogic relation is where there is a purposeful intention to initiate, modify, develop, or change knowledge, conduct, or practice (or all three) by someone who already possesses the knowledge and can evaluate it. Identities can be shaped and threatened by changes in the codes. For instance, students with pre-existing knowledge of healthcare and nursing understood some aspects of professional practice. When students had this knowledge, their identity as a learner diminished, and their identity as a worker increased. It also meant the midwife was no longer that student's teacher with respect to that practice knowledge and thus a different relationship was constructed.

7.2 Identity and relationships

Identity, according to Bernstein, refers to 'contemporary resources for constructing, belonging, recognition of self and others, and context management (what am I, with whom and when)' (Bernstein, 2000, p.205). Identity and relationships are always intertwined because learning how to be a midwife is a social process. 'What am I' can be understood by exploring the concept of classification, the relationships between boundaries. These can, as the code formula above states, be internal or external. 'With whom', can be explored by framing, the interactional practices within and between contexts. Framing considers the sequencing and pacing of learning and who controls this. Recognition of the context and the relationship, the 'when', is therefore essential to realise or demonstrate a legitimate text. These elements of the code will be explored in turn.

7.2.1 What am I?

'Classification provides recognition rules for both transmitters and acquirers for the degree of specialization of their text' (Bernstein, 2003, p.214). Where there is a strong classification the rule is that things must be kept apart (Bernstein, 2000, p.11). Conversely, where there is a weak classification, things are bought together. Power relations maintain the degree of insulation and the principle of classification. A strong classification has a unique identity, voice, and rules, while a weak classification has less specialised discourses, less specialised identities, and voice. Regardless of the classification, strong or weak, there is always a power relation, the regulative discourse. The power is often disguised; in this analysis, the aim is to show where this power lies.

Classification can be used to show boundaries between agents, discourses, practices, and contexts. The classification can be *internal* such as the relationship between agents and tasks *within* a context, or *external* between theory and practice or everyday knowledge and specialised midwifery knowledge, and *between* different practice environments.

7.2.2 Agents

Within the category of agents, I discussed transmitters and acquirers; there were various sub-categories depending on age, ability, and ethnicity; called sub-voices (Bernstein, 1990, p.26). Some students were school leavers, the difference in their age and the midwife's tended to be greater than mature students. The difference can be expressed as C+ for a significant age difference or strong classification and C– for similar ages and weak classification.

Students come to the midwifery course with varied educational backgrounds. This includes traditional A Level students with high tariff points, those with access courses, and several with previous degrees. Three kinds of students have already been identified, those with nurse first qualifications, those with informal healthcare knowledge, and those with no previous hospital or healthcare knowledge. The internal classification between students who were new to healthcare and their midwives would be considered C+, while the difference between a midwife and a nurse or healthcare worker might be C–. By the end of the course most students had a close pedagogical relation with their midwife, and thus the classification strength for these relationships was weak (C–).

Most of the students and midwives in the local area identified as White British; however, a few were from EU countries and two students identified as Black and mixed ethnicity, respectively. When students and midwives were from similar backgrounds, this weakened the internal classification between them (C–). When UK students were with EU midwives or vice versa, there was a strong internal classification (C+). This seemed to impede access to midwifery knowledge. The student cases presented in Chapter 6 were disproportionately from backgrounds other than White British. Of the seven cases presented, three were from 'other' backgrounds. Because the classification strength regulates power, some students, where there was a strong classification (C+), were inhibited to talk in front of their midwife, ask questions, or access learning opportunities. Whereas weaker classification (C–) enabled greater opportunity to discuss midwifery. It was this potential discourse that was available to be pedagogised that restricted or enabled access to meaning for students.

There was some sign of hierarchical positioning of students, with some nurses and midwives contemplating the 78-week students had greater status. However, this was not a universally shared perspective. It was interesting that some midwives who had undertaken the three-year course thought the 78-week students had greater knowledge, while other midwives foregrounded the experience of the three-year students. According to Bernstein (1990, p.26), positioning within categories or sub-sets is hierarchically arranged. However, it depended on whose position was considered.

The difference between the three types of students and their reactions to undertaking the clinical observations of blood pressure, temperature, and pulse was explored using external classification between the educational knowledge and everyday knowledge. Two types of students (78-week and previous healthcare workers) already had this knowledge. Thus, this can be understood as weak classification between their earlier everyday knowledge and the new midwifery knowledge. The students who found undertaking the observations positive for their developing midwifery identity had strong external classification; this activity was new to them. Therefore, students differed with respect to what knowledge they wanted to gain and whether they had any power in negotiating this. Dissatisfaction expressed by the former student types was in relation to no new learning and being part of the workforce rather than a student.

Many students wanted the internal strong classification to be weakened; this enabled a space for students to negotiate their learning. Finding common ground in mundane activities was one way of weakening the boundary, whether it was a slimming club or a shared professional status. The similarities between midwives and students, rather than differences, weakened the classification strength as the midwife identified with the student as comparable to one of them.

Midwives too differed in relation to 'what am I'. Midwife identities, like student identities, varied. Some were locally educated, others came from EU countries, and there was a range of educational qualifications, ages, and experiences. These sub-groups, like the students, can be categorised, and with each category a different discourse appeared. For instance, when midwives trained years previously, there was a strong external classification between their expectations and the students. Many midwives did not have a degree, and this separated their experience from the current students'. When midwives had qualified more recently, or they were currently studying the classification was weaker. Midwives identified with other 'conscientious midwives', a feature of internal strong classification and a shared identity. They distanced themselves from midwives they considered were less professional. Often strong classification was noted when midwives said they worked in an area they thought was more or less specialised than other midwives. The diverse discourses can also be arranged hierarchically, although the order of the hierarchy will change according to who orders them. For instance, midwives working on the birthing unit thought their work was the epitome of midwifery practice while midwives on the obstetric unit considered their work was more specialised. Students heard these discourses, and this affected their learning and the importance of skills and work in each area.

7.2.3 The discourses

Chapter 3 presented three specific discourses: communication is a natural skill; clinical skills are important; and evidence-based practice is not part of every midwives' work. When midwives documented that students were natural communicators, the message received by students was that this was not an area of practice they needed to improve. Students spoke of 'chatting' to women or their midwife and their terminology disguised the assessment of a woman or the feedback they received. Midwives were in a position that enabled them to elaborate the importance of communication skills in different contexts; however, few did this, perhaps because it was tacit knowledge or because they were busy. There were exceptions to this, and some types of midwives foregrounded communication skills, and role modelled exemplary forms. However, according to the students, these midwives were in the minority. Thus, the message projected by the profession was that midwives naturally have effective enough communication skills.

The significance students placed on activities and skills was also part of the discourse presented in Chapter 4. Being sent to the pharmacy was not seen as a symbolic learning opportunity. However, caring for a woman in labour was. The students talked about caring for women in labour for extended periods. Students justified undertaking these activities due to the understaffing in Trusts. Understaffing in midwifery was a contributory factor in unsafe and substandard care at Mid Staffordshire Hospital (Francis, 2013). Since the publication of the

Francis report, safer staffing levels have been advocated (NICE, 2015). However, there are challenges in practice which affect the provision of midwifery care, such as the rising levels of obesity, maternal age and complexity of care needed by some groups of women, and the shortage of midwives, estimated to be around 2600 (Paparella, 2016). Thus, student midwives despite their supernumerary status perceived that they were providing midwifery care.

When students cared for women in labour without drawing their midwife's attention to this or complaining, they were considered team players; this was documented in the PADs. However, when students asked for support, they were told by some midwives they needed to become more independent. The message received was clear: asking for support while caring for a woman in labour is not always a legitimate request. This was not a local issue; the RCOG (2018) Each Baby Counts progress report documented that student midwives nationally were caring for women without supervision.

Working within the limits as a student was reinforced by the midwives in the conversations they had with students but also in the feedback in the PAD. When students were 'trusted' to provide care to women, the message they received was that they were safe to practice. However, some students were not enabled to lead their own learning or called back from activities by a midwife, and this sent a different message. The activities students sometimes wanted to take part in were not seen as acceptable by the midwife, and the consequence was explicit midwife control.

Some students understood they were supposed to be learning as a student midwife but felt they were working as a qualified midwife. The boundary or degree of insulation between the two discourses: to *become* a midwife and *being* a midwife, should be kept apart (C+) but they came together. The weaker classification (C–) enabled students to build their professional identity as a midwife. This was reinforced when midwives mistook second-year students for third years and when women knew and used students' names and asked for them instead of a midwife. However, the interactional practices of not supporting the student may mean they had insufficient skills to provide effective care.

The degree of insulation is a regulator of the voice. Thus, the voice students could express in the practice was limited by their status. A change in the classification enabled a different voice to be heard. The more relaxed relationships between students and midwives in the community especially seemed to help a different voice to appear, one that enabled them to ask for more support or further clarification. Conversely, when students were noted to have concerns in practice, presented in Chapter 6, the classification between students and midwives tended to become stronger when ordinarily it weakened at the end of students' courses. This reduced the amount of space the student had to negotiate, and thus their voice was limited further.

The silent discourse or the omission seen in the data was the underpinning theoretical and evidence-based practice that supports the care midwives provide. These aspects of the curriculum were considered the work of the university and therefore not part of the discourse, except by a few midwives. These tended to be the midwives who had recently studied because they could see the relevance of this form of knowledge to practice.

7.2.4 The contexts

There was a strong classification between practice and education contexts. Students recognised these strong classification principles. The insulation between the placements was also strong, especially between hospital and community areas. Epistemologically the contexts were vastly different. Hospital knowledge differed from community knowledge, and hospital knowledge was afforded a specialised status that undermined some student's confidence. Acquisition of hospital knowledge was expressed as more important than community knowledge by students. The strong classification of the hospital environment, which was so different from their external 'normal lives' resulted in raised anxiety about the area. This is perhaps the difference between mundane/profane and esoteric/ sacred knowledge. Conversely, the knowledge demonstrated in the community was considered more common sense.

The difference between the contexts shaped a further discourse heard in practice. It seemed acceptable for students to be cautious of knowing enough in the hospital environment, and they repeated the discourse that several qualified midwives were apprehensive of working on CDS, especially. When midwives voice these concerns the message students hear is that CDS is a place to worry about. Students thought they had insufficient time on CDS to develop their skills. However, most of the students in this study had more time on CDS than in the community. It was not only the work, but the interactional practices on CDS that differed from the community, and this meant students worked with less direct supervision from their midwives. This potentially limited the students' learning and contributed to less practice knowledge in this area of midwifery practice which may have contributed to their worry.

This section has considered the 'what am I' dimension of identity construction; it has shown differences in students' internal and external classification. How some saw themselves as unprepared for midwifery while others had some or a great deal of experience with nursing or healthcare. Some students saw themselves as like other students, while others thought there were diverse types of student. The discourse of being or becoming a midwife is offered to show how student identity is formed and reinforced or hindered in pedagogic relationships.

The reason for the lengthy consideration of classification is that it is important to understand classification from internal and external perspectives to articulate variables with the pedagogic code. The identity of the student and midwife is the internal value, the way the person positions themselves, their dress and posture (Bernstein, 2003, p.14). External classification is the relations with others, the students' earlier life, and in this study to each placement. The principle of classification provides the means of recognising the agent and context and provides a voice.

7.2.5 With whom

Framing is *how* discourses are transmitted and acquired in pedagogic relationships, and with whom (Bernstein, 2000). Framing refers to the locus of control over the hierarchy, selection, sequencing, pacing, and criteria of the knowledge to be acquired. To be an effective transmitter, an elaborating code was needed. This involved a relationship: something was unpacked by someone; the process of making the meaning available to the acquirer. Midwives differed with respect to their pedagogic relationships: some preferred to be in explicit control of the student learning (F+); others were more relaxed (F–). Over time most student–midwife relationships weakened, especially in the community.

Students talked about relationships with midwives positively and negatively. This is a feature of other research, although Bernstein's framing codes are not used to label them. Midwifery mentors have been called guiding or controlling (Hughes and Fraser, 2011). The guiding midwives would be F– and controlling F+. Students in Hughes and Fraser's study and this one preferred less explicit midwifery control. Understanding the nuances, the invisible rules, maximised the students' chance of developing positive relationships with midwives and accessing midwifery knowledge. While the midwife's role was to enable students to move from outsider to insider status, much of this work was incumbent upon the students.

The status of the student is important because the internal classificatory value affects the interactional practices. Specific practices were acceptable or unacceptable for first-, second-, or third-year students. Differences were noted in behaviour, dress, demeanour, and acceptable speech patterns: the texts that were evaluated. The rules were about order, relation, and identity: the regulative discourse.

The first-year student midwife, in relation to a midwife, should behave in a certain manner. When the first-year student did not conform to their midwife's expected behaviour, they would be reprimanded. However, as the student progressed through the course, and the classification value weakened, it became harder for midwives to exert the same level of authority over students. The exception to this was when midwives recognised the difference between them and the students, at the end of the students' course, was greater than usual: strong classification when it should have been weak. The third-year student was not like a midwife and therefore the classificatory value altered. This change enabled midwives to refer a students' practice because the student's manner was 'unacceptable'. However, the change in relations was hard for all parties, and often caused student and midwife identity crises, as demonstrated in Chapter 6.

Midwives kept their power in the pedagogic process by reinforcing the regulative discourse. Bernstein (1990) calls this the pedagogic device. First-year students should recognise the symbolic boundary between the hierarchical relations in the hospital, especially, and respect these. However, it also meant first-year students could not ask too many or certain types of questions. The potential discourse available to some students was limited by some midwives. This was noted in one student's PAD, especially. The midwife wrote that the student was 'putting too much pressure' on herself by asking too many questions. When the midwife asserted her authority by writing this comment in the student's PAD. The pedagogic device influenced the student, and she appeared to stop asking questions which then further limited the potential discourse available to her. This in turn may have been what affected her ability to show sufficient midwifery practice knowledge.

The significance of the above section is the analysis of social relations, the practices, and message this sends to students. The form of control is described in terms of its framing. If the students understand the features of classification and framing, whether they are strong or weak, they are likely to be able to recognise and then realise the appropriate text. However, if they do not recognise them, they may be unable to realise the legitimate text. Students 'voice' what could be said in a particular context by recognising their status and the contexts boundary. However, what was said is the message; this is a feature of framing. The stronger the framing, the smaller the space for variation in the message. This means only certain things are permissible in this context. Thus, identity is not only developed in pedagogic relations but in the space available for variation. This is the voice–message relationship. This space can become a site for alternative realisations. This is the difference between thinkable and unthinkable knowledge.

7.2.6 When

The 'when' of this work is about the criteria for assessment. In any teaching relation, the essence of the relation is to evaluate the competence of the acquirer (Bernstein, 1990, p.66). Anything that can be evaluated is a criterion. This includes, conduct, manner, and the midwifery specific knowledge. Like the other rules, the criteria can be explicit or implicit. Most students recognised their behaviour was being observed, and that having the right attitude was essential for midwifery success, as Chapter 6 explained. Students who could not demonstrate the right amount of confidence or communication skills were not awarded high practice grades, and sometimes this affected their entry into the profession.

Midwifery specific knowledge was not always assessed sufficiently, especially when the midwife did not witness the student performance. Leaving students in the room happened more often in the hospital than in the community. Some students considered midwives would know they had met the criteria without observing the student undertake the specific skill. Others knew of strategies to ensure the criteria were visible to their assessors and reiterated conversations with women back to their midwives. Bernstein calls this phenomenon a realisation rule (2003, p.55) where the student 'selects interactional practice and text in accordance with recognition rule' – by this, he means this student recognised what she had to do to be seen and realise this rule.

Not realising the criteria came in many forms, some students were not able to show the legitimate text because they had not been taught or did not feel able to ask questions to learn. Others were unable to meet the expectation of their midwife; these students were either referred or left the programme. This could be interpreted as the dominant voice of the midwife silencing the student's voice. Some students still had a career to return to as a nurse. However, some students left towards the end of three years with an unnamed diploma in higher education and no professional career.

It is the recognition of the relation between a student and midwife and between types of knowledge that symbolises power and within the context that signifies control. In certain areas, and in certain relationships, some students are afforded some power and control; however, others are excluded from this. Midwifery research shows the hospital environment and senior midwives working in this structure used devices to keep their authoritative position (Hunter, 2005). I suggest we need a midwifery profession that recognises similarities to, rather than differences from, each other. It would help students learn how to be midwives and in their transition to qualified status and help create more supportive midwifery relationships.

The purpose of this section is to show the criteria for assessment in the midwifery profession are diverse. The rules of social order, conduct, character, and manner, embedded in the regulative discourse seemed to be assessed more than the specific midwifery knowledge. Messages are relayed to distinct groups of students that reinforce they belong or are excluded from the profession based on these criteria.

7.3 Midwifery knowledge is a vertical discourse

This section will explore types of midwifery knowledge to show that practice, using Bernstein's theory, is not commensurate with a graded performance. Midwifery knowledge may be hard for students to access initially. Access to meaning is through higher levels of elaboration and abstraction. Students may not recognise this knowledge until it is unpacked by a transmitter. Experts unpack this knowledge through formal pedagogies (elaborated codes) to enable access to this form of vertical knowledge. The assessment of this form of knowledge is through an exam of some kind and performances are graded in terms of ability (Moore, 2013). Midwifery practice at Sanderling University, and other universities across the UK, is not usually assessed by one formal exam. An ongoing record of achievement forms at least part of the assessment of practice based on observation and interactions in clinical practice between students, midwives, women, and the multidisciplinary team. Midwives assess student competencies throughout their education and sign to prove achievement of these in ongoing records or PADs. At Sanderling University, students' practice was summatively graded at the end of the year against set criteria. Thus, two forms of assessment were embedded within the assessment of practice: competence of specific skills and an end of year graded performance.

Bernstein uses the terms horizontal or vertical discourses to explain the separate ways for pedagogic transformation, and how knowledge is taught. He suggests this new language could enable a more productive and general perspective or lead to research possibilities and interpretations. I am using it to explore how students learn midwifery in practice. 'Horizontal and vertical discourses are seen as in opposition to each other', rather than complementary (Bernstein, 2000, p.155). One form may prosper at the expense of the other; one is oral while the other is written. In this way, one could differentiate midwifery practice, which is transmitted orally, from midwifery theory, which tends to be written. However, Bernstein goes on to say horizontal discourse is every day common-sense knowledge and vertical discourse is scholarly knowledge. As midwifery practice is not just common-sense knowledge but specialised knowledge drawing on many sources, both theoretical and practice knowledge, it is a form of vertical discourse.

Bernstein further differentiates between vertical discourses, using the terms hierarchical and horizontal knowledge structures. (It is unfortunate that Bernstein uses the terms horizontal in two separate ways and hierarchy for knowledge and relationships.) Hierarchical knowledge structures can produce knowledge, using higher levels of theory as in the university setting, while horizontal knowledge structures have limited ability to do so, such as in the field of practice.

7.3.1 Knowledge structures

Hierarchical knowledge structures are drawn as a triangle integrating propositions at higher levels of abstraction. The more hierarchical the knowledge structure is, the greater the emphasis on sequencing: some things must be taught before others for student learning. In the theoretical curriculum, normal physiology is usually taught before pathophysiology for the latter learning to make sense.

Horizontal knowledge structures require the learner to acquire and accumulate more specialised languages for each area of practice; there is less emphasis on the sequence in which this knowledge is taught. In midwifery practice, while it would be desirable for student's learning to reflect the theoretical pattern, moving from normality to more complex care, the sequencing of practice cannot be controlled in this way. Even though students typically start in practice areas considered able to facilitate normality, in the community and birthing unit, the first woman they meet may have complex care needs. The order of placements, whether students attend the community or birthing unit, does not affect their learning process, as students need exposure to both areas to acquire the specialised languages from each. Even though there may be some preference for one area of the other, the order is not as important as it is with hierarchical knowledge structures.

In Bernstein's code, the letter L is used to demonstrate horizontal knowledge structures, L_1, L_2, L_3. The L stands for the set of specialised languages necessary for each area. In this study, they can be considered the languages used in the community (L_1), in the birthing unit (L_2), and delivery suite (L_3). 'The set of languages of one area are not translatable to another area since they make different and often opposing assumptions, with each language having its own criteria for legitimate texts' (Bernstein, 2003, p.162). Students need to know which specialised language to use in each area of practice to demonstrate an authentic text.

The specialised language is acquired through oral transmission with midwives; a social interaction with those who already possess the appropriate 'gaze' (Bernstein, 2000, p.164). The gaze is the acceptable way of undertaking the practice in this setting using the hegemonic language. To relate this to my study, the language of the community or birthing unit reinforces the normal physiological processes of pregnancy and the postnatal period or birth, respectively, while, on the delivery suite, risk is the hegemonic language; thus L_1, L_2 and L_3. Using this theory, a different gaze is needed for each area.

In addition to this gaze, a particular style or specialised language was also needed for each midwife (L_5, L_6, L_7, etc.). Examining the student's PADs, three-year students had 7–11 different midwives assess their practice during their course. The 78-week students had six or seven. This meant each student may have had to acquire this number of separate gazes. I say may to illustrate that if the midwife was prescriptive, the student would need to acquire that particular gaze or way of working. If the midwife was flexible, there was room for negotiation on which gaze was adopted. However, the belief by many students was that learning their midwife's preferences was necessary to be considered capable of producing a legitimate performance. In this way, there is no one legitimate performance as each midwife, depending on their style and place of work has their own criteria.

7.3.2 Knower claims and authority

Bernstein (2003) makes one further distinction between horizontal knowledge structures: those with strong and weak grammars. Horizontal knowledge structures consist of a series of specialised languages (weak grammar) and a set of discrete languages for particular problems (strong grammars). The difference between the strong and weak grammars has been likened to the difference between the professions with medicine and law, seen as a strong grammars, and the professions of nursing, midwifery, and teaching, seen as weak grammars (Young, 2008). Moore (2013) makes a further point on this: he sees strong grammars associated with knowledge claims, whereas weak grammars are associated with knower claims.

This position echoes Hunter's (2005), where midwives are the knowers rather than midwifery as a knowledge-based profession. This means the midwife is the authority. The capital of knowers 'is bound up with the language and therefore defence of and challenge of other languages is intrinsic to a horizontal knowledge structure', particularly with weak grammar (Bernstein, 2003, p.162). The seeming lack of evidence used to inform midwifery practice and the need to know registrant's individual preferences can be interpreted to show midwifery practice as a horizontal knowledge structure with a weak grammar. From women's perspectives too, breastfeeding advice is seen as contradictory and knower dependent rather than informed by a strong grammar or evidence-based claim. Even though there is a plethora of evidence-informed breastfeeding knowledge to support women, how this knowledge is relayed appears to be different according to who offers it.

There is a resemblance between horizontal knowledge structures, particularly those with weak grammars, such as midwifery, and the horizontal discourse

(Bernstein, 2003, p.165). Both the discourse and knowledge structure are horizontally organised, and both are segmented. Acquisition of the horizontal discourse is tacit. It is taken to be understood implicitly. Hence, my initial confusion as to the nature of the discourse of midwifery knowledge transmitted in practice. Some students expressed the idea that midwifery knowledge was mundane or common sense. However, specific midwifery knowledge is embedded within common-sense knowledge. Examples to illustrate this are how to answer the telephone in hospital or whether to offer a woman a drink. The student must know something about the situation to respond appropriately to either example. Specific midwifery knowledge is needed as well as everyday knowledge in this context. To explain this, I revisit the horizontal discourse.

The horizontal discourse is every day common-sense knowledge. It is likely to be 'oral, local context-dependent and specific, tacit, multi-layered and contradictory across but not within contexts' (Bernstein, 2000, p.157). It is segmentally organised. What is acquired in one segment or context and how that knowledge is acquired may bear no relation to another. Thus, one can see how midwifery knowledge of the birthing unit is different from knowledge of the community or ward. The local environment and the specific type of care midwives provide can be contradictory between the placement areas. While the principles of midwifery care should transcend physical boundaries, there were 'them and us' divisions noted in practice between different midwifery areas. Students were acutely aware of these differences. How a woman is cared for in the latent phase of labour on a ward compared to a birthing unit may be very different, for example. Segmental learning is usually carried out in face-to-face relations, by implicit modelling or showing. The pedagogy is repeated until the competence is acquired. Note the use of the word competence; this form of knowledge cannot be assessed at higher levels: the student can either undertake the task/procedure/competence or not.

Bernstein goes on to explain how horizontal discourses have a repertoire of strategies available to the individual and a reservoir available to the community. Each member of the community uses some of the strategies within a reservoir of shared strategies. Where there is development of individual's repertoires, there needs to be sharing of practices. Midwives do not tend to work together in the same physical space; they work alongside each other in the community, visiting different women or undertaking clinics in separate rooms or hospital areas. They do, of course, discuss their strategies and can learn from each other. Students though, work very closely with their midwives often in a shared physical space. This enables a sharing of repertoires between each midwife and the student.

When midwives share knowledge with their student, there is a new set of strategies the midwife may adopt to expand her individual repertoire. The midwife's repertoire becomes available to the student's reservoir. Examples were also offered with regards to midwives learning from students sharing research knowledge. When individuals are isolated there is less development of the repertoire or reservoir. Some students recognised midwives who were more isolated and that this limited the development of their practice. Therefore, in horizontal knowledge structures with weak grammars, there can be many ways of demonstrating the appropriate text, but there are limited ways of creating greater generality and integrating knowledge as this is a feature of a hierarchical knowledge structure.

To add weight to the notion that horizontal knowledge structures with weak grammars cannot be graded a few more points are considered. Horizontal knowledge structures with weak grammars lack theory (Moore et al., 2013). While midwives, here I include myself, may not like this proposition, Rosemary Bryar, the author of the first textbook on theory for midwifery practice, recognised this. The need for the book came from a lack of theory for midwifery and was first published in 1995 (Bryar, 1995; Bryar and Sinclair, 2011). While there are now many theories for midwifery practice, they are not always used in practice; instead students learn theories in university.

The discourse about the lack of theory for practice, which many students and midwives seemed happy to share, was that they did not consider themselves academic. As a graduate profession, this creates a paradox. If midwives do not identify as academically inclined, the message they send to students is that theory, and perhaps evidence-based practice, does not matter. This is the pedagogical device; it is the force exerted on the curriculum from within the profession to control the status quo. It raises questions about who controls what. This contradiction, a graduate profession who does not value theory and research, reinforces the knower stance. It dichotomises midwifery knowledge.

Skilled midwifery care results from a combination of the personal qualities of the midwife with knowledge and theory (Bryar and Sinclair, 2011). The combination is the co-existence of the inner knowledge of the person, with the outer knowledge of the world. It is this strong relationship between the internal and external and empirical and theoretical that needs to be developed for midwifery knowledge to become a strong grammar. The combination of these forms of horizontal knowledge structures will lead to greater descriptive and explanatory powers.

Other authors suggest there could be some verticality (hierarchy) in horizontal knowledge structures (Maton and Muller, 2007; Young, 2008). In my research, some midwives, particularly M5 and M9, could alter the specific knowledge in their context of practice to aid student learning through problem-solving or the use of extreme examples. Both these midwives facilitated this activity for students through reflective discussions. This gave a greater orientation to meaning for students. Instead of students learning in front of the woman, either through observation or practice, these midwives used the space outside the clinical room or in the car for learning. This meant more of the midwife, and her knowledge, was available to the student.

If there is some verticality in horizontal knowledge structures, there may be a differentiation of knowledge. By this, I mean, pass and excellent categories for assessment. However, this verticality was not seen in all midwives' interviews. I asked each midwife how they taught and assessed knowledge, and many found this question hard to answer. This could be due to how I asked the question, because not all midwives facilitate verticality or because midwifery practice knowledge was tacit and therefore difficult to articulate. Midwives knew how

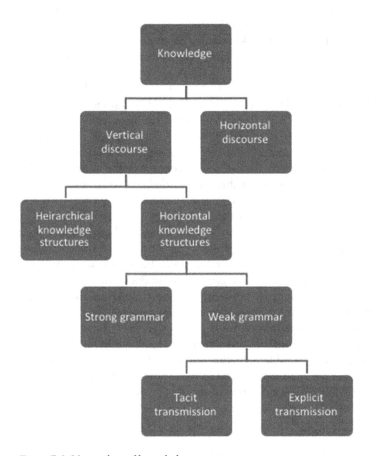

Figure 7.2 Verticality of knowledge structures.

to care for women but not how to elevate the learning to a more abstract level. Therefore, I suggest not all students are given access to this more hierarchical form of practice knowledge (see Figure 7.2).

Lastly, horizontal knowledge structures with weak grammars, languages, or approaches tend to displace or vie for power rather than complement each other (Moore et al., 2006). This can be exemplified by the discourses between theory and practice and how, if a student is practical, this counts for more than theoretical knowledge for students and midwives alike. Other examples in this case study included one CDS midwife who spoke of the 'fast pace' and different expectation of students in her environment compared to community or birthing unit. While she did not say one area was better or worse than another, it was implicit within her comparison that some areas were more lenient on students, whereas she expected more.

The nature of knowledge in midwifery practice is only part of the problem relating to grading student's practice. The relationship between the student and midwife is pivotal. Midwifery knowledge is transmitted in the instructional discourse, but this is always embedded within the regulative discourse (Bernstein, 2003). This means that midwifery knowledge is secondary to the hierarchy between the student and the midwife. Thus, the knower is more important than the knowledge.

This interpretation resonates with midwifery education research in another area of the UK (Hunter, 2005). Hunter studied 27 midwifery students from both courses and ten hospital-based midwives; she noted students had to base their practice and personal style on that of their mentor. This was felt most acutely by the students on the shortened course. She concluded midwifery was a 'practitioner-based' profession, whereas nursing was 'context-based' (Hunter, 2005, p.258). This case study suggests that midwifery knowledge is both a practitioner-based and context-based profession, with specialised languages for both the placement area and the individual midwife.

When midwives reinforced to students in their PADs to 'be yourself', it was not just an encouraging comment but a positive evaluation of the students' character. Be yourself praises the person, not the action. The trouble with this form of feedback is that it is unspecific. The general praise does not explain to the student what about their manner is positive. The way to improve the feedback would be to explain how an interaction with a particular woman was positive, so the student can reflect and learn from this.

To bring the discussions from the earlier chapters together and show how they relate to grading practice, a table depicting strong and weak classification and knowledge structures has been constructed to show how the Bernsteinian terms (in bold) link to midwifery learning and assessment (Table 7.1).

7.4 What does this mean?

The concepts of classification and framing have been applied to midwifery students and their midwife's experience of teaching and assessing in the clinical environment. Now, the exegesis of Bernstein's theories needs to be explored to consider what this means in relation to assessing and grading midwifery students' practice.

At the start of the midwifery course, there is a strong classification between students and midwives, between ordinary knowledge and midwifery knowledge and the difference between individual midwives' practices and the contexts. If the midwife is in explicit control of the student's learning activities, the pacing and sequencing of midwifery knowledge and the criteria for assessment, features of strong framing, the pedagogy is visible to the student. According to Bernstein, the output of these modalities C+/F+ is a graded performance where the underlying rule/principles are 'things must be kept apart' (Bernstein, 1977, p.120).

However, there are differences in types of students, and this can affect the relationship and orientation to meaning with midwifery knowledge and with their midwife (C−). Some students are enabled to lead their own learning, and this is accompanied by a weaker framing relation (F−). This form of pedagogy is

Table 7.1 Bernsteinian concepts and their relationship with midwifery

		Strong/explicit/visible pedagogy	*Weak/implicit/invisible pedagogy*
Classification (what/voice/ power/ instructional discourse and recognition rules)	Agents	Student–midwife: The difference between the agents, especially in the first year, is vast. Student–woman: strong classification at the end of education as the student is more like the midwife than the woman.	Student–mentor: The difference between many of the students and their midwives in the third year is reduced as students share the workload and have socialised into the profession. Student–woman: difference weak at the beginning of students' education.
	Discourses	Evidence-based practice and research are the students' work. **Hierarchical knowledge structure** Students who know when to ask for help can be trusted because they are safe.	Students and midwives have a 'natural ability' to communicate with women. **Horizontal knowledge structure**
	Practices	Difference between individual midwives' practices is vast, examples given, hands on or off the perineum, is noticeable. Similarly, how midwives offer information to women (and students) is variable.	Principle of woman-centred care, rather than individual preference shapes practice. Multiple ways of knowing.
	Contexts	Difference between each area. What happens on delivery suite is different from the ward or MLBU or university.	Once students understand the principles of midwifery care the differences between the contexts are less noticeable, except CDS, it seems which retains its special status. This is reinforced in midwives' discourses too.

(Continued)

Table 7.1 (Continued) Bernsteinian concepts and their relationship with midwifery

		Strong/explicit/visible pedagogy	Weak/implicit/invisible pedagogy
Framing (how/ message/ control/ regulative discourse and realisation rules)	Hierarchy (order, character, and manner)	Midwife in charge. Higher status. The student should be willing to work, enthusiastic. Not challenge the midwife, especially at the beginning of their education.	Professional friendship develops Later, students can join in 'gossip'.
	Sequence/ pace	Normal midwifery first. Need to have hands-on experiences to learn. Midwife decides if student 'ready' for opportunities.	Student has increased ability to negotiate experiences. Less control from the midwife.
	Criteria	Emphasis on what is absent from product against explicit specific criteria. **Performance model**	Emphasis on what is present in the product against implicit diffuse criteria Regulative discourse likely to remain explicit. **Competence model**

invisible. When this happens (C–/F–) the assessment modality is one of competence assessment. The student knows and recognises when they have produced a legitimate text.

In certain areas, the hospital and delivery suite especially, the classification between everyday knowledge and this world of work is still strong (C+). There seemed to be a clear division of labour between some students and the midwife (C+), as some students talked of providing midwifery care without direct and sometimes limited indirect supervision. Other students talked of teamwork, where the classification was weaker (C–). The ability of some students to negotiate extra support was limited; thus, the framing style of some midwives could be described as strong (F+). Others felt supported (F–), although there was often hesitation about the level of support on CDS. Therefore, both assessment modalities; competence and performance models could be used in the hospital depending on the interactions between the student and mentor.

This could explain the variation of feedback for students on CDS. Some students could navigate the system and request feedback, or they worked with a midwife who fostered positive relationships with others, and she offered this. However, other students had no voice to request this. They were excluded from feedback on their performance in this area, and this limited students' access to midwifery knowledge. Not supplying feedback is one way some midwives may maintain control of the specialised midwifery knowledge, even though this may not be deliberately withheld.

The time spent with the midwife in the hospital was often episodic. The fast-paced environment meant there was little time for explanations for care decisions and individual midwives practices needed to be learned for student success. Students did not always think the midwives saw enough of their practice to accurately assess the student's performance. In addition, the nature of knowledge in clinical practice has limited verticality; thus, the ability to differentiate it at higher levels of abstraction is reduced.

The emphasis on performance models is what is missing in this product. Many students had confidence missing on CDS. In the hospital environment having a nurturing midwife was important, yet it was often in the community that students said the reciprocal relationships developed. In the community, the relationship between the midwifery specific knowledge and everyday knowledge was less noticeable (C–). The relationship between the student and midwife was also more relaxed (C–), which enabled the student to direct their learning (F–). The student–midwife dyad had more time together. It was not just the relationship but the continuity, which enabled the students to develop confidence, which was missing in the hospital.

Achieving skills, no matter how small, had a positive effect on a student's confidence. When midwives gave students positive feedback, it made a difference. Confidence is an internal and external condition, which develops through feeling a sense of belonging, in the relationship with the midwife and by participation in practice. It works on an individual and social level. When students did not get a sense of belonging or a connection to a midwife, they were often unable to show sufficient knowledge, but this was often bound up with confidence. They were then at risk of being referred in practice and leaving the profession.

As midwifery practice is based on the idea of woman-centred care, where the woman is central, and her concerns and decisions must be bought together, I argue the assessment modality midwifery practice needs is a competence model. This principle fits better with midwifery than a performance model where the underlying rule/principles are 'things must be kept apart' (Bernstein, 1977, p.120). However, with a competence model, the regulative discourse criteria of conduct and manner are likely to be more explicit. This was seen in some of the student cases presented in Chapter 6. Midwives judged students on their attitude despite not all being good role models themselves. Attitudinal concerns need to be shared with students earlier to enable them time to develop and embody more professional behaviours. Equally, midwives have a professional duty to role model professionalism.

Furthermore, the criteria used to grade practice are underdeveloped and not shared by all (transmitters and acquirers). There are multiple interpretations of grading midwifery practice across the UK (Fisher et al., 2017). The criteria used to assess performance are neither explicit to all learners nor shared by all assessors, yet they need to be if a performance model is used (Bernstein, 2000, p.44). The lack of specific grading criteria was not just noted at a local level.

The Lead Midwife for Education (LME)-UK scoping study, in which I was part of the research team, explored grading midwifery students' practice and determined that the timing, individuals involved, components, and credit weighting varied (Fisher et al., 2017). Therefore, there were inconsistencies across the UK. The conclusion of this work said that grading was considered more robust and meaningful than pass/refer and that midwives were positive about the value given to practice and their role as gatekeepers of the profession (Fisher et al., 2017). I have mixed thoughts about these collective findings now.

At Sanderling University, I do not believe grading student's practice was more robust than the earlier competence assessment of practice. Grading expressed whether students recognised and realised the rules of their midwife. It encouraged students to be compliant with the established orthodoxy. The grades carried meanings about whether the student was accepted. Thus, it also signified those who were not. Student cases presented in Chapter 6 show discrepancies between qualitative and quantitative feedback and grades. This suggests some midwives had difficulty discerning differences between performances, and some may have been reluctant to perform their gatekeeping role. I do not think the experiences of the students and midwives in this study are unique and therefore question whether grading of practice for all students is more robust.

The criteria for competence have been clearly stated by the NMC (2009) in the domains of practice and Essential Skills Clusters, and more recently in the six domains of the new standards of proficiency for midwives (NMC, 2019). While there are discussions about how these are interpreted, I question whether midwifery education needs both assessment modalities, competence assessment, and a graded performance, based on my data and the literature. The midwifery profession needs a practice assessment that combines the personal qualities of care, empathy, and communication skills with underpinning knowledge and evidence-based practice (Renfrew et al., 2014). Observation of students' practice alone is unable to measure all these elements, especially when the midwife is not always present when students communicated with women and other members of the multidisciplinary team. Oral examinations may enable a more rigorous assessment of midwifery knowledge, and this aligns with the oral tradition of horizontal knowledge structures. It also has the capacity to foreground knowledge from the knower.

While Bernstein's distinguishes between competence and performance, as outputs appearing from recognising who I am, in relation to whom and where, these distinctions are not shared by all theorists. Others see the assessment of performances to inform judgements about ongoing competence (Norris, 1991). These judgements are generalisations about the likelihood that the student will be able to be professional and practise safely in the future (Norris, 1991).

7.5 Changes affecting the code

From this research, I am suggesting grading students' practice at Sanderling University based on observations of their clinical care was neither a robust nor trustworthy assessment of the students' practice. The usually close relationship between students and midwives at the end of the students' course, lack of time, absence of explicit theory, or research from practice decisions and nature of observation undermined the midwives' ability to accurately grade students' practice.

The relationship between the midwife and student was central to learning midwifery practice and essential for pastoral support. However, the dual roles of supporting and assessing the students may have created tensions for midwives (Bray and Nettleton, 2007). Practice learning could not always be prioritised, and this affected the students' ability to access practice knowledge. The nature of observation meant the underpinning rationale for midwifery care, and orientation to meaning was not articulated by the student, and thus the midwife was only able to judge the student's practice on what they saw.

Recently, new models of practice learning have been introduced into nursing and midwifery practice arenas. Collaborative Learning in Practice (CLiP) and Practice Education Based Learning: Suffolk (PEBLS) are models where two or three students learn from each other facilitated by a coach rather than in a one to one relationship with a mentor (Lobo et al., 2014; HEE, 2014). The coach is not needed to combine clinical responsibilities with teaching; their role for the shift is to facilitate student learning. The organisation and the philosophy underpinning student-led and peer-facilitated learning is patient-centred, with the students providing care supported by the coach. There is a greater emphasis on knowledge and evidence underpinning care and students have structure to their learning, including an hour of protected learning time to research the patients' condition and care needs. The care is analysed and presented back to the coach and peers, thus increasing the students' communication skills too. Evaluations so far have been positive from students, staff and patients.

However, this model is not a panacea, and it may only be viable in limited areas of midwifery practice. To date, students have had opportunities to learn on the antenatal and postnatal wards and some clinics using this model, but having junior students learning from more senior students in the presence of a midwife in birthing areas or women's homes may not be woman-centred or practical.

The reliance on the relationship between the midwife and student to access practice knowledge is reduced in this model as students learn with and from one another, often with other year groups. This potentially enables greater access to midwifery knowledge as first-year students can ask a second year a question they might not ask a midwife as the classification is reduced. Midwifery knowledge, evidence, and communication skills are foregrounded in this model and, therefore, when this is embedded within the midwifery curriculum students' practice could be graded daily, with explicit feedback to improve their performance. The likelihood is that student performances will be stratified as distinct types of learners, and the knowledge they possess will be more visible. Students and midwives value the practice environment for learning and want this aspect of the students' performance reflected in the degree qualification; therefore, there is potential in this model not only to better differentiate between student performances but also to raise midwifery knowledge within the profession. However, it may not be possible in all areas, and the areas students may want the greatest access to midwifery knowledge are unlikely to be able to support this.

The Council of Deans for Health discussion paper (CoDH, 2017) suggested the NMC revisit the rationale for grading of practice or a pass/fail assessment informed by the evidence base. The evidence base includes the 'grading of practice in pre-registration midwifery' project, a national study undertaken by and on behalf of the Lead Midwife for Education United Kingdom Executive (LME-UK), including myself. The research was conducted over five years, in three phases. The first was a scoping study which identified variations across the UK of grading practice noting challenges in achieving consistency for midwifery students (Fisher et al., 2017). The second was a set of grading principles which were developed using a Mini-Delphi approach (Fisher et al., 2018). Eleven consensus statements were agreed from participants of the group. The final phase developed a generic framework for practice assessments with a toolkit for midwives to support the feedback they offer to students, whether as an assessor or supervisor (Fisher et al., 2019).

The NMC have revisited this pedagogic decision in their latest standards (NMC, 2019). There is no mention of whether practice is graded; that decision is up to each university to make when it adopts the new standards by 2022. This is appropriate because the NMC is a professional regulator, not an educational establishment. However, it is likely to introduce more variation to midwifery curricula again as some universities will retain grading of practice and others move to competence assessment.

The CoDH (2017) also suggested a national midwifery assessment tool may help reduce the inconsistencies and have clearer criteria against which all student midwives are assessed. Across England and Northern Ireland, Midwifery Practice Assessment Collaboration (MPAC) created a new midwifery practice document. The document is for students across the two countries commencing their studies on curricula approved against the NMC (2019) *Standards of Proficiencies for Midwives* under the NMC (2018) SSSA framework. This document, welcome as it is, has the capacity to be used with a graded performance or competence assessment.

7.6 Recommendations

One of the recommendations of this research was to separate the role of the mentor as a midwife who teaches and nurtures students in midwifery practice from their assessment role. In 2018, the NMC Standard for Student Supervision and Assessment was published, which did just that. Three separate roles are now stated: practice supervisors, practice assessors, and academic assessors (NMC, 2018). The practice supervisors will be responsible for orientating students to their learning outcomes and supporting them to gain practice knowledge. They will share their assessment of the student's practice with the practice assessor. This person will confirm the achievement of student learning in conjunction with the academic assessor. A more robust assessment of student competence and/or performance could be achieved with attention paid to the variables that seem to enhance or corrupt practice assessments. However, with the practice assessor further removed from the student, another discourse is likely to be heard.

Furthermore, the quality of learning will still be affected by the relationship between the student and practice supervisor and time available in clinical practice for learning. If the model of learning and assessment in midwifery changes to the CLiP or PEBLS type, this may enable greater access to practice knowledge and the evidence base for students in some areas. Students will be responsible for delivering woman-centred care, supported by a coach. They will be able to learn and develop the clinical skills they currently value but will also need to demonstrate decision making and a sound understanding of the woman's history and condition. This has the potential to elevate midwifery knowledge in clinical practice.

A further recommendation was that the number and types of skills students are expected to demonstrate should change to meet the expectations of the role of the midwife. This has also happened with the publication of the NMC (2019) standards of proficiency for midwives. These are based on evidence about midwifery as a profession, including a framework for quality maternal and newborn care (Renfrew et al., 2014). The importance of interdisciplinary conversations and education are foregrounded to enable recognition of each other's contribution to care for women and babies but also to raise standards. As midwifery students qualify against these standards, further research will need to be undertaken to see if this transpires.

When these standards (NMC, 2019) are implemented, they will, like the NMC (2018) standards, have implications for students and midwives as they affect the pedagogic code. Already, I envisage some midwives wary of the change and increase in knowledge that students need to demonstrate. Midwives caution will come from several possible positions, including skills they may not possess themselves. As this book has shown, Bernstein offers a language with which to examine these changes in terms of classification and framing and their effects on the pedagogic code.

7.7 Reflections, strengths, and limitations of this study

The analysis of this case study is influenced by my own background, values, and experiences. I am aware of these as potentials for bias. I share the language code of midwifery with the participants, which meant I had the potential to understand their meanings; however, I might not have recognised nuances and new phenomena. Similarly, prior to becoming a midwife, I was a nurse, this means I may have interpreted the 78-week programme more positively than the direct entry course. Any research undertaken by a single researcher can result in limited perceptions. Not only was I the instrument for data collection, which has advantages and disadvantages, I interpreted the data too. I decided what was included and excluded, and I had the authority to do this; however, I thought reflexively about each decision.

The knowledge presented in this case study may not be complete, as the data was collected over a period of several years, and I did not know initially what I was looking for. Rigour in the analysis would have been aided by having an independent assessor to discuss the concepts. To overcome these shortcomings, I included diverse opinions from others and discussed this work with my academic supervisor and peers; one of these was a direct entry midwife.

The use of Bernstein's theories as a conceptual framework as well as axial codes may have limited the analysis of the data. I was purposely looking for his concepts. However, I recognise that his code theories can only partially explain how students learn in clinical practice. Not only are the nuances in student–mentor relationships too varied, but they are also too complex to be fully explained. His theories are generated from observations of education in schools; the primary purpose of these institutions is to teach students. In clinical midwifery practice, the primary purpose is to care for pregnant women, teaching students is secondary to this and, as the case has shown, executed to varying degrees of success. However, his theories have been used by others in vocational and higher education and in practice settings to good effect (Muller et al., 2004).

A further weakness of this work is in limited links with other theorists. Bernstein also displays limited relation to other scholars other than Emile Durkheim, Karl Marx, and George Herbert Mead (Atkinson, 1985). Although Moore (2013) says he also drew on Weber and symbolic interactionism and many other traditions, but these are the only ones he lists. To balance this weakness in my research, a wide range of professions as well as midwifery specific educational research has been critiqued and included in the book.

At the start of the research, I was a junior member of the midwifery team with a close relationship with the students. I taught them often, they saw my performance, and I made this more visible to them by highlighting weaknesses in my knowledge or presentational style. For instance, I said, I may have been a practising midwife, but I have never thought of that, or I am not sure I fully understood that concept. I also remember saying, the order I presented it could have been more logical. When this happened, I tended to use the opportunity to research the concept in class with the students present, thereby role modelling learning together and showing the students how and what knowledge to access to link theory to practice. I did not mind reflecting on my teaching practice in front of them and evaluating my teaching performance. I think this enabled the students to confide in me and take part in my research.

As time progressed, I came across fewer unfamiliar concepts, and my presentations improved; thus, I had fewer opportunities to reflect on my performance to share with the students. I knew how to answer their questions in class. The distinction between me as a novice teacher and the students as novice learners had changed. Using Bernsteinian terms, the classification between them and I had altered from weak to strong. This distance and time may have helped my analysis of the data.

My identity as a researcher changed too. I am no longer a novice researcher and have contributed to more than my own work on grading practice (Fisher et al., 2017, 2018; 2019; Way et al., 2019). I have more knowledge and confidence in my ability to contribute to curricula developments and conversations about professional identity. Although I also recognise that I am not an expert.

Contending with the ethical tensions of this work has been an ongoing struggle, and that has enriched my understanding of case study method, research practices, and assessment of students' practice. I can explore the relationship between the means of gaining knowledge and the knowledge obtained. Initially, I thought there should be a relationship between students' theoretical grades and practice; especially with those struggling to write an academic assignment nevertheless awarded high practice grades. The paradox of this was that I considered myself a 'good' midwife, yet my post-registration degree classification was 2:2. Therefore, my ability to express theoretical ideas and be a midwife could be, according to Bernstein, strongly classified. Now I appreciate that theoretical knowledge does not need to be communicated in written form only to be a good midwife, but it does need to be present and communicated orally for the profession to move from a knower to knowledgeable status.

I feel my work could be transferrable to other midwifery students' experiences and that collectively as a profession midwives ought to explore the nature of midwifery knowledge. Whether it is a horizontal knowledge structure with weak grammar and what that says about the identity of midwifery as a profession. A strong grammar is associated with knowledge claims, while a weak grammar is associated with knower claims. While midwifery is a unique profession, its identity and voice could be strengthened by foregrounding what is known from who knows. Engagement with the *Lancet Midwifery Series* (Renfrew et al., 2014; RCM, 2018) has the potential to support this change. Similarly, there are opportunities to engage with the ongoing development of professional identity as the content of the midwifery curriculum across the UK is amended to meet the NMC (2019) standards and further evidence based publications are produced by the professional body, the RCM. Collectively, the unique identity, voice and rules of the midwifery profession can be elevated to become a horizontal knowledge structure with a strong grammar. This in turn has the potential to better support women with evidence based care.

7.8 Summary

I have shown there is a strong classification between knowledge gained in the university and the practice arena; each has a unique quality of otherness. Student identities develop from recognising the rule of the specialised discourse or practice in each context, so then they can realise the legitimate text or performance. The legitimate text in practice differs from the university expectations.

Early socialisation into the profession by a supportive relationship with a midwife is needed for students. The lack of relationship with a midwife, especially in the first stages of their education left some students feeling they had limited access to learning midwifery. Some midwives were better at explaining midwifery practice to diverse groups. These groups and their differences were explored.

The community environment and midwifery-led birthing units, to a lesser degree, tended to have weak classification and framing strengths between students and midwives. In these environments, the midwives had a relaxed relationship with students; the workload was mostly about normality, with opportunities for reflective practice and discussion. Students were often able to select learning opportunities and develop competence.

Conversely, working in other areas of the hospital, the ward and CDS, the classification and framing was stronger. Students typically had less control in these areas. They were allocated to care for women according to clinical workload rather than student choice. Midwives tended to be more directive in these areas, and the pace of the work meant there was more emphasis on completing tasks. In the hospital, the student's practice was considered less visible to the midwife. The workload was sometimes divided, and the student and midwife each had their role. Each midwife's differing practice, especially in the hospital, needed to be learned for students to feel they could demonstrate the legitimate performance of that registrant.

With such differences in strengths between classification and framing, one would expect different outputs of students. However, the outputs were generally the same, a high practice grade. This was regardless of the tool used, practice area, differences between the students, or midwives. The conclusion is that grading midwifery practice in its current form, based on observation, is neither robust nor trustworthy. This undermines the credibility of the practice grade and devalues the currency of midwifery student's degree classifications. As a profession, midwives need to demonstrate evidence-based care, effective communication, and affective domain skills and theory. We need to ensure all these aspects of the role of the midwife are assessed and move from a knower profession to a profession which values knowledge equally.

Bibliography

Bernstein, B., (1977). *Class, Codes and Control Volume III.* 2nd ed. London: Routledge.

Bernstein, B., (1990). *Class, Codes and Control Volume VI The Structuring of Pedagogic Discourse.* London: Routledge Taylor and Francis Group.

Bernstein, B., (2000). *Pedagogy, Symbolic Control and Identity Theory, Research, Critique.* 2nd ed. Oxford: Rowman and Littlefield Publishing Group inc.

Bernstein, B., (2003). *Class, Codes and Control Volume 3 Towards a Theory of Educational Transmissions.* 2nd ed. London: Routledge and Kegan Paul Ltd.

Bray, L. & Nettleton, P., (2007). Assessor or mentor? Role confusion in professional education. *Nurse Education Today,* 27(8), pp. 848–855.

Bryar, R., (1995). *Theory for Midwifery Practice.* Basingstoke: Palgrave Macmillan.

Bryar, R. & Sinclair, M., (2011). *Theory for Midwifery Practice.* 2nd ed. Basingstoke: Palgrave Macmillan.

CoDH, (2017). *Educating the Future Midwife – A Paper for Discussion.* London: CoDH UK-Wide Future Midwife Advisory Group.

Fisher, M., Bower, H., Chenery-Morris, S., Jackson, J. & Way, S., (2017). A scoping study to explore the application and impact of grading practice in pre-registration midwifery programmes across the United Kingdom. *Nurse Education in Practice,* 24, pp. 99–105.

Fisher, M., Bower, H., Chenery-Morris, S., Galloway, F., Jackson, J., Way, S. & Fisher, M. M., (2018). *Report on Final Phase: National On-Line Survey (Phase 3 of the Grading of Practice in Pre-Registration Midwifery Project)*. United Kindom: LME-UK Executive.

Fisher, M., Bower, H., Chenery-Morris, S., Galloway, F., Jackson, J., Way, S. & Fisher, M. M., (2019). National survey: Developing a common approach to grading of practice in pre-registration midwifery. *Nurse Education in Practice*, 34, pp. 150–160.

Francis, R., (2013). *Report of Mid Staffordshire NHS Foundation Trust Public Inquiry*. London: London Stationery Office.

HEE, (2014). Practice Education Based Learning: Suffolk (PEBLS) Coaching as a *Teaching and Learning Strategy*. Cambridge: NHS Health Education England.

Hughes, A. J. & Fraser, D. M., (2011). There are guiding hands and there are controlling hands': Student midwives experience of mentorship in the UK. *Midwifery*, 27(4), pp. 477–483.

Hunter, B., (2005). Emotion work and boundary maintenance in hospital based midwifery. *Midwifery*, 21(3), pp. 253–266.

Lobo, C., Arthur, A. & Lattimer, V., (2014). *Collaborative Learning in Practice (CLiP) for Pre-Registration Nursing Students*. Norwich: UEA.

Maton, K. & Muller, J., (2007). A sociology for the transmission of knowledges. In: *Language, Knowledge and Pedagogy; Functional Linguistics and Sociological Perspectives*. London: Continuum.

Moore, R., (2013). *Basil Bernstein the Thinker and the Field*. Abingdon: Routledge.

Muller, J., Davies, B. & Morais, A., (2004). *Reading Bernstein, Researching Bernstein*. London: Routledge Farmer.

NICE, (2015). *Safe Midwifery Staffing for Maternity Settings*. London: National Institute for Health and Care Excellence.

NMC, (2008). *Standards to Support Learning and Assessment in Practice*. London: Nursing and Midwifery Council.

NMC, (2009). *Standards for Pre-Registration Midwifery Education*. London: Nursing and Midwifery Council.

NMC, (2018). *Standards for Student Supervision and Assessment*. London: Nursing and Midwifery Council.

NMC, (2019). *Standards of Proficiency for Midwives*. London: Nursing and Midwifery Council.

Norris, N., (1991). The trouble with competence. *Cambridge Journal of Education*, 21(3), pp. 331–341.

Paparella, G., (2016). The State of Maternity Services in England. Oxford: Picker Institute Europe.

RCM, (2018). *State of Maternity Services Report 2018*. London: Royal College of Midwives.

RCOG, (2018). *Each Baby Counts Progress Report*. London: Royal College of Obstetricians and Gynaecologists.

Renfrew, M., Homer, C. S., Downe, S., McFadden, A., Muir, N., Prentice, T. & ten Hoope-Bender, P., (2014). *The Lancet Series on Midwifery Executive Summary*. London: Lancet.

Way, S., Fisher, M. & Chenery-Morris, S., (2019). An evidence-based toolkit to support grading of pre-registration midwifery practice. *British Journal of Midwifery*, 27(4), pp. 251–257.

Young, M., (2008). *Bringing Knowledge Back in: From Constructivist to Social Realism in the Sociology of Education*. London: Routledge.

Appendix 1
Grading practice literature search strategy

Search strategy hits and chosen articles. Several combinations of key words were used to maximise the literature search. Truncation of the terms grade* or grad-ing* was used to ensure all the variants and plurals of words would be captured (Ridely, 2008). Student* or undergraduate*was used as a second search string to encompass the change to an all graduate profession but also other professions already at graduate level such as physiotherapy. 'Practice' or 'clinical practice' or 'professional practice' was searched with the near to proximity locator. The database searches were conducted with the support of a subject librarian to ensure rigour and relevancy.

A further search string for evaluat* OR measure* OR assess* OR fail* OR apprais* OR perform* Or competen* was used as these terms were frequently seen in the international literature. However, when combined with the Boolean operator AND this search limited the number of hits significantly and excluded much of the relevant literature. When used with OR it increased the search significantly but not the specificity of the sources. Thus, after several weeks of searching to find the most effective strategy which was precise enough to prevent the retrieval of too many irrelevant papers and sensitive enough to find relevant sources, the final search strategy included three search strings combined with AND. One further search was used to exclude literature which included child* or adolescen*; however, this was only available in two of the databases (CINHAL and ProQuest). Papers were required to report empirical research if the data was gathered from or about grading students' clinical practice.

Search 1 – Grade* OR grading*
Search 2 – Student* OR undergraduate*
Search 3 – Practice OR clinical n2 Practice OR professional n2 practice
Search 4 – combine S1, 2, and 3
Search 5 – child*or adolescen*
Search 6 – Search 4 NOT search 5

Limiters were set to include English language only, dated from 2000, within academic journals.

Table A1.1 Grading practice literature search strategy

CINHAL Grade* OR grading* (51,032) Student* OR undergraduate* (155,812) Practice OR clinical n2 Practice OR professional n2 practice (439,062) Combine S1, 2, and 3 (894) child* OR adolesc* (762,948) S4 NOT S5 (416) 2000 (361) 2000–2017 (288)	Health and medicine (14 databases)	Medline via UEA – 1576 hits	Google Scholar
1 (Docherty and Dieckmann, 2015)	(Donaldson and Gray, 2012)	(Eggleton et al., 2016)	(Scammell et al., 2007)
2 (Smith, 2007)	(Imanipour and Jalili, 2016)	(Lawson et al., 2016)	
3 (Oermann et al., 2009)	(Briscoe et al., 2006)		
(Andre, 2000) – opinion but oft-cited	(Susmarini and Hayati, 2011)		
4 (Dalton et al., 2009)	(Hanley and Higgins, 2005)		
5 (Heaslip and Scammell, 2012)	(Meldrum et al., 2008)		
6 (Walsh and Seldomridge, 2005)	(Manning et al., 2016)		
7 (Roden, 2016)			
8 (Hatfield and Lovegrove, 2012)			
9 (Pulito et al., 2007)			
10 (Murphy et al., 2014)			
11 (Lurie and Mooney, 2010)			
12 (Plakht et al., 2013)			
13 (Fisher et al., 2017a)			
14 (Seldomridge and Walsh, 2006)			
15 (Hiller et al., 2016)			
16 (Edwards, 2012) Isaacson – opinion Roberts-performing arts – opinion			
17 (Paskausky and Simonelli, 2014)			
18 (Fazio et al., 2013)			
19 (Weaver et al., 2007)			
20 (Scanlan and Care, 2004)			
21 (Amicucci, 2012)			
22 (Lefroy et al., 2015)			
23 (Clouder and Toms, 2008)			
24 (Manning et al., 2016)			
25 (Reubenson et al., 2012)			

Table A1.2 Literature search table

Author and date	Country	Sample size	Design	Data collection	Analysis	Findings	Comments
Not counted							
(Helminen, 2016)	Finland	23 articles reviewed	Literature Review on competence mainly	Ke words, inclusion criteria presented, but no search stings to replicate the study. 725papersfound, 37 screened 23 relevant to the review	Methodological and country of origin classification then thematic analysis	Three themes based on the timing of events prior to, during and after assessment process- last theme very short. Many subthemes. Common assessment practices are rare, so mentors need to familiarise themselves with the process. Most schools offer pass refer assessments, with fewer offering graded scales with three, four, or five levels. Usually assessed by observation with accompanying questioning. Disagreement	Not explicitly related to grading except that fewer of the included studies graded practice and 3-5- level scale. Inconsistency a common theme

(Continued)

Table A1.2 (Continued) Literature search table

Author and date	Country	Sample size	Design	Data collection	Analysis	Findings	Comments
						as to whether written assignments can assess practice. Helpful student traits influence the assessment. Mentors tend to avoid negative feedback to students. Lack of courage to fail students	
Isaacson Roberts			Opinion Opinion- performing arts				
Andre 2000	Australia	Not stated	Debate-opinion piece supported by literature but no details of search terms/inclusion or exclusion criteria	n/a	n/a	Seems in favour of grading for practice based courses. Says the move to higher education and to value practice it should be graded. Challenges the notion that subjectivity	% in upper 25th centile. Authors said it decreased grade inflation, but it is still present

Not counted
Not counted

Not counted

(Continued)

Table A1.2 (Continued) Literature search table

Author and date	Country	Sample size	Design	Data collection	Analysis	Findings	Comments
						does not render the assessment invalid. Rationale for grading comes from employer with a suggestion that 35% of grade comes from this. However, if all students typically get high grades I am not sure the employer will be able to discern the average from the exceptional and some failing students might be due to negative interactions in practice and not their ability	

(Continued)

Table A1.2 (Continued) Literature search table

	Author and date	Country	Aims	Sample size	Design	Data collection	Analysis	Findings	Comments
34	(Dalton et al., 2009)	Australia and New Zealand	Develop and refine a national grading tool for physiotherapy	Pilot 1 university 295 students Filed 1: 9 universities/ 747 students Field 2: 9 universities 695 students Inter-rater reliability testing five universities 30 student educator pairs	Action research project to design and test a grading tool	Interviews (n=9 clinical educators), Focus groups (eight in pilot with 4–14 participants), surveys and training sessions (four in pilot with 14–25 participants)	Statistical analysis for survey Qualitative data analysis for interviews and focus groups by independent research assistant. Checked by project team member	17 minutes to assess a physiotherapy student. Most educators 90% found the performance indicators comprehensive Students positive (no % given) large standard deviation as to whether mark reflects performance, some felt they deserved better scores. Others were a reasonable summary of performance. Wanted a wider range than just four descriptors. In test site 2 it took 28 minutes to grade. Inter-rater reliability was high. DVD examples provided for educators of exemplary performance	

(Continued)

Table A1.2 (Continued) Literature search table

	Author and date	Country	Sample size	Design	Data collection	Analysis	Findings	Comments
33	(Weaver et al., 2007)	3349 evaluations, 1612 before the card changed, 1737 after	A more explicit grading scale decreases grade inflation in a clinical clerkship.	Evaluated change of daily shift card evaluation	Before and after study, hypothesising more explicit criteria would reduce grade inflation in medical education	Altered from shift care H/high pass/pass/fail to five choices upper 5%, upper 25%, expected, below expected or far below	Descriptive statistics	Before change honours 22% HP 49%, pass 28.4% fail 0. After change upper 5–9.8% upper 25% 41.2% expected 46% below 2.8% far below 0	1 Interventions should be developed to address grade inflation and failure to fail
32	(Fazio et al., 2013)	USA	Grade Inflation in the Internal Medicine Clerkship: A National survey	To determine extent of perception of grade inflation	National survey 64% response rate of clinical directors in north American medical schools	questionnaire	Descriptive analysis	55% agree grade inflation exists. 78% report it as a serious/ somewhat serious problem and 38% note students who should have failed have passed	
31	(Smith, 2007)	UK	14 midwifery mentors from 30 volunteers (five mentors with degrees and two working towards masters so stratified sample) all graded between 3–10 students	Explore midwives experiences of assessing and grading student midwives			Four themes emerged from the data analysis – clinical competence versus academic ability, ability to award an academic grade, the grading process and the social process of assessment	Mentions safe practice Friends Fitting in Happy talking pass/fail less so grades Social factors have potential to affect the grade

(Continued)

Table A1.2 (Continued) Literature search table

	Author and date	Country		Sample size	Design	Data collection	Analysis	Findings	Comments
30	(Meldrum et al., 2008)	Ireland	To investigate inter-rater reliability in physiotherapy on a standard graded assessment	N=86 paired physiotherapy student assessments with two educators (one practice tutor and one practice educator). Eight tutors and 50 practice tutors	Inter-rater reliability study	Grading sheets	Inferential statistics	Two grades agreed on 74% of occasions (n=64). The most common grade disagreement was between a 2:1 and first (n=11), then 2:1–2:2 (n=9) and finally 2:2–3rd(n=2). The mean difference in marks was −0.5 with actual marks within 6.2 of each other. this demonstrated a high level of reliability.	Students on placement 4–6 weeks. Assessment form three sections, patient management (marked out of 600), professional development (marked out of 300) and organisation for third year (100 marks). Each of these further broken down into 36 criteria. Form available but not scoring protocol. Study was appropriately powered.

(Continued)

Table A1.2 (Continued) Literature search table

	Author and date	Country	Sample size	Design	Data collection	Analysis	Findings	Comments
29	(Walsh and Seldom-ridge, 2005)	USA	To examine the relationship between theory and clinical grades	N=184 nursing students' grades	Comparison between theory and practice grades	Student grades for ten paired theory and clinical courses	Descriptive statistics	Clinical grades were higher than theory grades. The quality performance for a psychomotor skill was considered easier to judge than a client interaction. Some students did not have the opportunity to demonstrate all skills, yet faculty still reluctant to award lower grade due to no opportunity	Because clinical grades are awarded at the end of a placement the bias of recency may affect the grade, i.e. only recent behaviours are graded. Poor performance at the beginning of a placement may prevent the student getting an A but is unlikely to be failed. Suggestions to improve include multiple assessments (like medical students)

(Continued)

Table A1.2 (Continued) Literature search table

	Author and date	Country	Design	Sample size	Data collection	Analysis	Findings	Comments
28	(Murphy et al., 2014)	Canada	To assess feasibility of a new grading system	Convenience sample of 63 clinical educators for physiotherapy	Cross sectional survey to compare two grading tools for physiotherapy practice	Questionnaire to 63 CE 71 student grades students assessed at mid-point and end of placement using one of two assessment tools, new tool had 24-point assessment instrument covering four areas professional behaviour, safety, communication and patient management. Fail, weak pass, pass or exceptional	descriptive statistics	The PT-CPI of 51 students found 74% of student grades were good, 26% exceptional. Compared to the APP scoring 7% adequate, 52% good and 41% excellent. The APP score was quicker than the PT-CPI score and some scores in the latter were marked n/a	Need for speed when grading students is vital, yet does this reduce the quality of the feedback, become a tick box exercise

(Continued)

Table A1.2 (Continued) Literature search table

	Author and date	Country		Sample size	Design	Data collection	Analysis	Findings	Comments
27	(Susmarini and Hayati, 2011)	Indonesia	To explore clinical facilitators experience of grade inflation	Purposive sample of Six Nurse clinical facilitators from six schools	Qualitative, exploratory design using phenomenological method	Interview	Thematic analysis	Causal factors, the institution, faculty, students and education system. Lack of time, expectations of students and employers and the university affected the grade. Lower grades make students unsatisfied and can affect course evaluations	
26	(Scammell et al., 2007)	UK	To explore student mentor and education staff experiences with a grading practice tool	Nursing students 70, mentors 10, and educators 20	Qualitative approach research	Nine audio recorded Focus groups	Thematic analysis	Valuing practice-central theme, tripartite nature of practice learning, depends on good mentoring relationships, learning environment – some unprofessional behaviours seen – previous experience not always helpful – some mentors not enthusiastic using the tool	Difficulty recruiting mentors. Diagram on p25 good Many recommendations

(Continued)

Table A1.2 (Continued) Literature search table

	Author and date	Country	Aim	Sample size	Design	Data collection	Analysis	Findings	Comments
25	(Lefroy et al., 2015)	UK	To understand the meaning of feedback with and without grades	110 (76%) of 144 students volunteered, 24 declined randomisation, 4 changed their minds. 86 medical students were randomised to have grades and then no grades in weeks 1 and 2; however, only 83 finished. Of these, 83 most chose to have grades on their third and final assessment. 78% chose grades, 22% not	Realist evaluation cross over design. 24 were interviewed, 15 with grades and 9 without on final assessment	Questionnaire and accompanying grade or comments, cross referenced to order of randomisation and whether graded as borderline previously and gender	Coding and consensus between the two authors	Most students chose to receive grades. Students who chose to receive grades perceived them as representing additional information on their position and progress. The opposite of this argument was made that focussing on grades rather than content of feedback. There was mixed motivation from the grades. They could galvanise or reduce effort. Many students said they were in supportive relationships, but not all. To others grades	Grading scale must improve – borderline – proficient – very good. The four-week placement scores are calculated on week, 1, 2 and 4

(Continued)

Table A1.2 (Continued) Literature search table

	Author and date	Country	Sample size	Design	Data collection	Analysis	Findings	Comments
							represented a risk of harm. Some students ignored their borderline grades and focussed on the comments instead	
24	(Clouder and Toms, 2008)	UK	To explore the validity of assessment strategies specifically the clinical reasoning viva in physiotherapy	55 in total. Purposive sample, randomly selected. 18 final year physiotherapy students, 19 educators (range of experience from 18 months to 8 years) and 18 university tutors	Qualitative methodology of students, clinical educators and university tutors	One to one semi structured interviews. Pilot study resulted in minor changes to the interview schedules	Grouped statements, themes, and triangulation	To determine if both assessments were necessary by all students and assessors thought the two assessments observation and clinical reasoning viva were essential. However, you needed to get along with the assessor, the CVR could be prepared some thought the CVR was tougher than	Very good introduction critique miller's pyramid

(Continued)

Table A1.2 (Continued) Literature search table

	Author and date	Country	Sample size	Design	Data collection	Analysis	Findings	Comments
								other universities assessments. CVR mark could differentiate between good and confident and high flying students. Considered the validity of the assessments. stakeholders
23	(Scanlan and Care, 2004)	Canada	To investigate the extent of grade inflation in Canadian nursing programmes	4500 clinical nursing grades	Case study method including retrospective analysis of grades i the faculty of nursing during the past 25 years	High school grades on admission, Cumulative GPA, clinical course grades	to compare school and undergraduate grades, relationship between grades in nursing and other professional programmes, the role of clinical grades to overall GPA	The grades for school and undergraduate study showed as parallel relationship. Grade inflation is identified in the nursing programme but also across the university, but to a lesser degree.

(Continued)

Table A1.2 (Continued) Literature search table

Author and date	Country	Sample size	Design	Data collection	Analysis	Findings	Comments
						90% of grades B+ and above, 60% of grades A or A+. in the final practicum, 80% of the clinical grades were A or A+. only 3% of students received a B or lower. These grades contribute significantly to the problem of grade inflation.	Not attending to grade inflation in nursing and midwifery programmes sends the message that student's performances meet high-level standards, when they do not. The credibility of the profession is at stake

(Continued)

Table A1.2 (Continued) Literature search table

	Author and date	Country	Objective	Sample size	Design	Data collection	Analysis	Findings	Comments
22	(Briscoe et al., 2006)	USA	To learn more about the nature, perceived virtues and deficiencies of the clinical grade evaluation	85 from 129 clerkship directors in medical schools offering psychiatry clerkships (66% response rate)	survey	26 item questionnaire	Descriptive analysis	Most universities had a mix of narrative and graded elements. Attendings graded students 100% of the time. Half the sample used fail/pass/ honours system (47%), 18% had a numeric score 32% had percentage/ letter, pass/fail only comments only or other. Most grading forms had been recently created or revised, suggesting the process is frequently in a state of flux. 65.2% assign a weighting of 50–70% of the overall grade to the clinical assessment. The justification that this stands to	Measurements include attitude, professional behaviour, interpersonal skills, communication, clinical skills, clinical knowledge Asking clerkship directors to answer a question on behalf of their attendings (without directly asking the attendings) brings in a source of error. The three most wanted evaluations are of clinical skills, professional behaviour and clinical knowledge,

(Continued)

Table A1.2 (Continued) Literature search table

Author and date	Country	Sample size	Design	Data collection	Analysis	Findings	Comments
						reason because it involves direct observation could be challenged. Despite the findings mirroring other medical research most respondents 88% indicate agreement or strong agreement that grade inflation is a problem. 20–30% of students awarded the highest grades, represent grade inflation. There was low confidence in the ability of attendings to discriminate between weak, failing and excellent students. The grading form may not measure	with interpersonal skills, communication and attitude less favoured. This was contrary to the survey's findings where the latter were considered very useful 25–35% of the time

(*Continued*)

Table A1.2 (Continued) Literature search table

	Author and date	Country	Sample size	Design	Data collection	Analysis	Findings	Comments
			To explore students experiences of a new grading tool					what psychiatry supervisors think should be measured. More education for evaluators was thought to help in 50% of the time, but 18% thought nothing would help grade inflation
21	(Hanley and Higgins, 2005)	Ireland	25 students invited 18 agreed to participate; however, only 11 took part, 5 to individual interviews and 6 to focus group. All students registered nurses, 3 had degrees, 2 diploma and itu experience from 0 to 10 years	Descriptive exploratory design (qualitative)	Semi-structured interviews and a focus group interview	Coded, compared, merged, themed	Language of clinical assessment tool (lack of focus and understanding), assessor differences issues of inter-rater reliability and need for assessors to spend more time observing students practice, Benner's level, mixed views (experienced	

(Continued)

Table A1.2 (Continued) Literature search table

	Author and date	Country	Sample size	Design	Data collection	Analysis	Findings	Comments
			Evaluation of timing of feedback from practice shift evaluations				staff constrained by not having all levels available to them), action plans and minimal use of portfolio. Interpreting the criteria requires deconstruction to identify its meaning. Recommendations modify language of assessment tool	
20	(Hiller et al., 2016)	USA	47 medical students, 547 times by 46 residents and attendings' end of shift evaluation	Quality improvement project to review all clinical shift evaluations. To determine of a delay in end of shift evaluation affects overall grade	Evaluation score, from student and assessor and date of shift and evaluation.	Descriptive and inferential statistics. Delay in evaluation was calculated. Immediate evaluation was 0–1 day, within the week 2–7	97% completion rate. Evaluations took a mean of 8.5 days to complete. 18% completed in 1 day, 28% within 2 days. Timing had no significant effect on score. Most evaluations	End of shift evaluation based on energy/ interest, knowledge, problem solving, clinical skills, personal effectiveness and systems based practice

(Continued)

Table A1.2 (Continued) Literature search table

Author and date	Country	Sample size	Design	Data collection	Analysis	Findings	Comments
					days and more than a week 8+ days. Power analysis undertaken and study well powered. Early and late evaluation compared across first and fourth week	completed in one week (56%), evaluators who had the most students were frequently later than those with fewer. 76% of students had all 12 completed, 1 student had only 9, the rest approx. 22% had 10/12. Most students 95% had at least one evaluation delayed by a week and one third by a month. There was more delay later in the quarter and student grades were slightly lower. Time data was missing on 12% of forms	Limitations, no analysis of qualitative comments, although anecdotally, as one would expect there were more comments the earlier evaluations submitted

(Continued)

Table A1.2 (Continued) Literature search table

	Author and date	Country	Sample size	Design	Data collection	Analysis	Findings	Comments
19	(Plakht et al., 2013)	Israel	124 nursing students	Questionnaire	students evaluated their	Inferential statistics.	Three findings:	Grade awarded by
		To evaluate the level of feedback and relationship to self-assessment, clinical performance and skills		All students received verbal feedback from at least two teachers daily lasting 5 minutes with a mid-point 15–30-minute comprehensive feedback session. Feedback was positive, negative and conclusions. Teachers tried to balance + and	feedback from teachers, the contribution of practice to their skill development and performance and the grades were also collected. Accuracy of student self-evaluation was measured against the teachers' grades		student's grades, accuracy of these and contribution of practice. Confounding variables included demographics and previous education and teachers. Measures of reduce self-performance, accurate and over presented. Teachers grades ranged from 65–100 with a median of 93%, most student grades were lower with a mean difference of -1.07 +/- 6 points. Most (60%) were	2–3 teachers and feedback offered daily, seems a strength of this study. Making time for quality feedback is essential. The ethnicity of students was compared with the majority (93.5%)being Bedouin, the minority seemed to have a significantly lower grade, however this was not reported in the findings

(Continued)

Table A1.2 (Continued) Literature search table

Author and date	Country	Sample size	Design	Data collection	Analysis	Findings	Comments
						deemed accurate with 25% undergirding themselves and 15% over grading. Students ranked practice contribution as very high. High-quality negative feedback can help students accurately self-assess, high-quality positive feedback can cause the student to overestimate their performance. Underestimation of performance was no associated with positive or negative feedback. Psychological factors may affect this. Students wanted constructive criticism to progress	

(Continued)

Table A1.2 (Continued) Literature search table

	Author and date	Country	Sample size	Design	Data collection	Analysis	Findings	Comments
18	(Edwards, 2012)	UK	38 midwifery student clinical grades	Evaluation of level 6 student grades (one cohort) from four assessments on application of knowledge. Students were assessed across five different maternity units	Average of practice marks compared to award for academic achievement in the practically based OSCE and Viva assessment of underpinning knowledge	Descriptive analysis, Standard deviation	Clinical grades were clustered0 which was according to the authors suggestive of consistency. Only 5% fell outside this range. While no statistical analysis was undertaken, Edwards considers this statistically significant. However, the point of the significance is not articulated. The average 'academic' grade measured by the viva or osce was much lower, which again was considered statistically	Edwards questions how mentors are assessing knowledge, rather perhaps the students' ability to perform tasks is being assessed rather than knowledge. (redfern suggests this). Which Edwards considers acceptable as midwives need to be able to perform care but she does acknowledge the profession is all graduate and students should be

(Continued)

Table A1.2 (Continued) Literature search table

	Author and date	Country	Sample size	Design	Data collection	Analysis	Findings	Comments
							significant but no statistics were offered. The differences were hypothesised to have come from the assessment tools and differences in the grading criteria, rather than a link between assessments	able to demonstrate underpinning knowledge of the evidence
17	(Paskausky and Simonelli, 2014)	USA	Evaluate relationship between exam and practice grade.	281 students on maternal childbearing course	Descriptive correlation study evaluated the relationship between exam style and final faculty assigned clinical grade for undergraduate nursing students	Two measurements collated. Clinical grades awarded using rubric. Students rated on professionalism, and communication skill, acquisition of clinical judgement. Exam 100 question multiple choice	Descriptive statistics	Exam showed normal distribution curve 59–93%, clinical grades skewed from 80–95%, with 90% higher than B+. Faculty assigned grades were higher in 98% of student grades. Only two students had higher grades on	Grading tool attached

(Continued)

(Continued)

Table A1.2 (Continued) Literature search table

Author and date	Country	Sample size	Design	Data collection	Analysis	Findings	Comments
						exam and one had the same for both. Over 90% of students (n=255) had clinical grade of 5 or greater in practice, nearly 70% had scores of 10 or greater and 18% had scores of 20 or greater. Therefore, the authors conclude grade inflation occurred due to low to moderate correlation between the two measurements and negatively skewed distribution and reduced range of faculty grade compared to exam.	

Table A1.2 (Continued) Literature search table

Author and date	Country	Sample size	Design	Data collection	Analysis	Findings	Comments
						There is an expectation that students with low exam scores should have a correspondingly low practice grade as practice is hypothesised to be underpinned with knowledge. Walsh and Seldomridge question whether there is a relationship between theoretical knowledge and competent practice or the validity of the educational evaluation methods. Therefore, the validity must be challenged. The possibility low exam results pose a threat to patient safety and the profession was postulated	

(Continued)

Table A1.2 (Continued) Literature search table

	Author and date	Country	Sample size	Design	Data collection	Analysis	Findings	Comments
16	(Manning et al., 2016)	USA	Evaluate new grading tool	Pharmacy students	Survey of students, n=67, preceptors n=106 2010 n=49 2014 and faculty but no results for faculty	5 point Likert scale Questionnaire and student grades	Descriptive statistics	Students were accepting of a move from needs improvement, acceptable, shows strength scale, to F/P. preceptors thought students would lack motivation, but this did not happen. Only 16% of students identified grades as the biggest motivator with most 47% desiring proficiency instead. Preceptors found assessing the students less challenging 18% with P/F compared to 35% for graded	The honours grading system impacted upon the students' grades, returning to p/f reduced their average gpa with no detrimental side effect and less student stress

(Continued)

Table A1.2 (Continued) Literature search table

	Author and date	Country	Design	Sample size	Data collection	Analysis	Findings	Comments
15	(Pulito et al., 2007)	USA	To determine if some performance characteristics are more associated with overall grade than others	Evaluation of Clinical performances of students conducted over two years	211 medical students evaluated by 2–3 faculty preceptors; total 585 evaluations- six students excluded because they scored lower than a B	Clerkship evaluation form used to evaluate students on ten descriptors using 5 point scale	Intraclass correlation, avova and logistics regression	395 (68%) received A grade, 190 (32%) B grade. Six evaluations excluded. No statistical difference between the two and four-week evaluation. Inter-rater reliability low between performance ratings and grade between 20–86 difference. Little to be gained from using multi-item forms professionalism +knowledge sufficient to obtain grade could use one of either oral presentation, clinical skills or diagnostic	Grading grid presented. Needs improvement =1, expected level −3, outstanding performance =knowledge, ability, skills, professional-ism, interper-sonal skills +(10 points) My interpreta-tion if we use knowledge and diagnostic ability + professional-ism this might help reduce grade infla-tion. However study sug-gested five items only needed

(Continued)

Table A1.2 (Continued) Literature search table

	Author and date	Country	Sample size	Design	Data collection	Analysis	Findings	Comments
							ability. The items rated highest were personal characteristics= such as interpersonal skills or professionalism, middle communication skills- oral and written, cognitive abilities and diagnostic ability lowest	
14	(Reubenson et al., 2012)	Australia	Seven examiners	Examine the agreement between multiple assessors in physiotherapy. To measure inter-rater reliability of physiotherapy student assessments examiners watched videoed examination and treatment of one patient from one student. They independently graded the student on five performance categories	The five individual performance scores and the overall grade of the seven examiners	Frequency analysis no statistical analysis	Variety in examiners grades spanning two or three grades. Scores ranged from 40-70. The global grade 5 mark was considered good with 5/7 examiners rating a similar grade (less than 50%), the other two examiners	Evidence of grade inflation, although not stated in the article

(Continued)

Table A1.2 (Continued) Literature search table

Author and date	Country	Sample size	Design	Data collection	Analysis	Findings	Comments
						awarded scores of 65 and 70%. 2/7 is a big difference with such a small group who were experienced with 8 years' assessment experience. The PPPA form consists of five performance categories: subjective examination; physical examination; analysis and planning; intervention and management; and professionalism (communication and documentation). For each category	

(Continued)

Table A1.2 (Continued) Literature search table

	Author and date	Country		Sample size	Design	Data collection	Analysis	Findings	Comments
								examiners are required to assign a grade (fail, pass, credit, distinction or high distinction) that best reflects the student's performance. Examiners are guided in their marking by a rubric	
13	(Eggleton et al., 2016)	New Zealand	To measure inter-rater reliability of GP grading tool	100 GPs	Not stated. GPs watched a video of student performances and graded from poor to very good	Four components: history taking, physical exam, clinical judgement and humanistic qualities. Distinction – 4, pass – 3, borderline pass – 2, or fail – 1.	Intraclass correlation coefficient to see if inter-rater reliability	Good reliability grades – however, a wide range of marks given. These grades were lower than usual clinical practice grades – possibly due to nerves of filming or because student not known to GP. Comments on untidy hair affected score. One outlier who graded	Statistics cannot measure this. The borderline pass student scenario was scored fail by 71%, borderline by 20% and good by 7%. Lower grades than usual thought o be due to no relationship with the student and the nerves of the filming/ exam process

(Continued)

Table A1.2 (Continued) Literature search table

	Author and date	Country		Sample size	Design	Data collection	Analysis	Findings	Comments
12	(Amicucci, 2012)	USA	To explore the experience of grading for faculty	11 faculty	Phenomenological using the framework power as knowing participation in change (Barrett 1988, 2010)	Interviews	Van Manen's approach	Five themes. Clinical grading is subjective. Classroom grading is black and white whereas clinical grading is grey. Considered the friends and family test- would I want this person caring for me. Safety was the benchmark and students could progress if there were no glaring safety issues. Opportunity to change, akin to benefit of the doubt, assigning fail grades is stressful. wishful thinking, a theme that	Helpful – some of my participants though grading was quite straight forward but these were mentors in practice not faculty, who had taught the student so concerns about how their teaching impacted upon student progression may influence this.

(Continued)

Table A1.2 (Continued) Literature search table

Author and date	Country	Sample size	Design	Data collection	Analysis	Findings	Comments
						meant different ideas to participants – most hoped for student improvement. The last theme was discontentment and disappointment with a variety of factors, student effort, and colleagues or administration support. Blending clinical and theory grades was a way for improvement	

(Continued)

Table A1.2 (Continued) Literature search table

	Author and date	Country	Sample size	Design	Data collection	Analysis	Findings	Comments
11	(Heaslip and Scammell, 2012)	UK	Evaluate a local practice assessment tool	107 nursing students (51% response rate), 112 mentors (86% response rate)	Two-stage mixed methods evaluation; stage 1 qualitative approach which gathered perceptions of the grading tool and helped develop a questionnaire that was circulated more widely	Questionnaire based on key themes of qualitative data		62% of Mentors felt confident grading practice but 67% wanted more education. 75% said the tool facilitated assessment of practice; however, the students thought the grades were unfair and varied hugely. Mentors thought they delivered effective feedback 92% but students only received it 56%. Similarly 89% thought the feedback matched the grade from mentors but students only replied yes 60%. Qualitative data suggested mentors valued grading practice some lacked confidence in failing students.	Excerpt of grading tool included – they separate unsafe from refer; pass (40–51%). Good pass 52–68%), very good pass 69–85%), excellent above 86%). Team noted practice grades skewed higher than previously, before grading

(Continued)

Table A1.2 (Continued) Literature search table

	Author and date	Country	Aim	Design	Sample size	Data collection	Analysis	Findings	Comments
10	(Docherty and Dieck-mann, 2015)	USA	To assess evidence of failing to fail	Cross-sectional descriptive survey	84 faculty responded (33% response rate)	37 item questionnaires	Descriptive and inferential analysis	88% said they were confident in determining clinical grade; however, 66% said they had worked with students who should not have passed. 72% admitted giving students the benefit of the doubt. Faculty did not feel supported to fail students. Rubrics were positive and negative. Evidence for failure to fail across the nursing school	Surprising how many admitted not failing a student, despite low response rate

(Continued)

Table A1.2 (Continued) Literature search table

	Author and date	Country	Sample size	Design	Data collection	Analysis	Findings	Comments
9	(Imanipour and Jalili, 2016)	Japan	Develop and evaluate a comprehensive assessment tool for nursing	38 students and eight instructors	Survey	Questionnaire to elicit views of new assessment. To analyse clinical skills two assessment methods were used global rating and Direct Observation Procedural Skill	Descriptive statistics	87% or instructors and 89% of students thought the new assessment was positive for learning. Satisfaction was high for both groups. Discussion based on the methods of assessment and why new tools align better with learning	
8	(Seldomridge and Walsh, 2006)	USA	To evaluate student grades for practice	204 nursing student grades	Not stated	204 student grades	Not stated – descriptive statistics	Very high grades awarded for practice. Most students awarded A or B. reasons why offered. Suggest multiple methods used and rubrics might help	Excerpts of grading tools/ rubric for behaviour from two assessments- medication administration and teaching project. Latter not nursing practice. *(Continued)*

Table A1.2 (Continued) Literature search table

	Author and date	Country		Sample size	Design	Data collection	Analysis	Findings	Comments
7	(Lawson et al., 2016)	USA	To characterise national assessment practices in medicine	172 clinical directors contacted. 58% agreed to participate n=100	Prospective cohort study	33 question survey	Descriptive and statistical analysis.	Clinical assessment tool used for 95% of participant's assessments	
6	(Lurie and Mooney, 2010)	USA	To explore variability of shift score cards and weighting for total grade	83 Medical students'	Statistical analysis of the student's grades from exam and clinical performance to assess bias	Student grades over five placements and exam results	To determine whether weighting of exam to clinical practice would affect overall grade	No evidence of bias between placement grades	
5	(Roden, 2016)	UK	To explore the impact on clinical grades on overall degree	1057 student occupational therapy grades	Audit to compare pre-practice marking and post-practice marking grades on overall academic averages	37–48 item criterion referenced practice report. Band A–F awarded by practice educators	446 student grades before practice marking were compared to 593 post-practicegrading	Each student received higher practice marks in each subsequent placement. The year 1 grades ranged from 60–68%, year 2 64–69 and year 3 67–72%. The authors conclude there was year on year inflation, level by level inflation and clinical versus academic grade disparity	One university but good number of students

(*Continued*)

Table A1.2 (Continued) Literature search table

	Author and date	Country		Sample size	Design	Data collection	Analysis	Findings	Comments
4	(Fisher et al., 2017a)	UK	To explore application and impact of grading practices in UK	40/55 LME (73% response rate)	Descriptive evaluation survey	questionnaire asking for the range of tools and practice assessment methods across pre-registration midwifery programmes	Thematic analysis	The findings were categorised into: 1) The process of grading practice; 2) The impact of grading of practice on mark profiles; 3) Clinicians' views on grading of practice. Wide UK variation despite NMC requirement. Most universities noted a rise in grades. Clinicians valued grading practice and there was some suggestion that over time more of the grades were used	Asked about clinicians' views on grading but did not ask clinicians, therefore there is a level of interpretation between LME responders and what they think clinicians' experiences are

(Continued)

Table A1.2 (Continued) Literature search table

	Author and date	Country	Sample size	Design	Data collection	Analysis	Findings	Comments
3	(Donaldson and Gray, 2012)	UK	To explore issues with grading practice	119 published articles	Systematic literature review	Database searches	Extracted data thematic analysis	Grade inflation, barriers and challenges, validity and reliability and mentor support and preparation. Low level of evidence – rubrics suggested to be a resolution	when their search strategy was replicated, it did not have same outcome – however, it is seven years later. Rubrics on search strategy, some literature included not focussed on grading. Six qualitative papers stated but only five found and two not on grading

(Continued)

Table A1.2 (Continued) Literature search table

	Author and date	Country	Design	Sample size	Data collection	Analysis	Findings	Comments
2	(Hatfield and Lovegrove, 2012)	UK	Evaluation of local grading tool	171 questionnaires 65 returned (38% response)	Development of (paper 1) and audit (paper 2) of a level 6 grading tool for practice. Graded on Professional conduct 15% Performance of a skill 35% Knowledge and comprehension 35% Reflection and evaluation of practice 15%	questionnaire	Not stated but? thematic	The professional conduct criteria were considered too broad by one assessor. Marks for practice were generally higher than theory. The authors said this can be expected in a practice profession but should this assumption be challenged. One participant questioned whether knowledge should be assessed in a practice assessment. 50% of Assessors thought students could not accurately self-assess – 15% said the students	Used in post reg critical care – yet still assessors thought students – qualified staff unable to assess their performance and grades higher than theory.

(Continued)

Table A1.2 (Continued) Literature search table

	Author and date	Country	Sample size	Design	Data collection	Analysis	Findings	Comments
							under-assessed with 9% of assessors saying students over assessed. 97% of assessors said they were prepared for their role	
1	(Oermann et al., 2009)	USA	To describe how faculty evaluate students and identify trends and grades in nursing nationally	Survey of 1573 prelicensure nursing pro-grammes' assess-ment and grading practices.	Web-based national survey 29 items including demographics and evaluation strategies used in clinical courses	Web-based questionnaire	Not stated? thematic	Observation of the predominant strategy (93%). Written assessments, skills testing, student contributions, conferences, self-assessment and simulation (45%). Most (83%) used pass/fail rather than graded clinical practice. Faculty evaluated student's clinical practice (87%) each time they were in the clinical setting. 98% used a clinical evaluation tool	

Appendix 2
Participant information sheet

Grading midwifery practice

Sam Chenery-Morris

I would like to invite you to take part in this research study. Before you decide I would like you to understand why the research is being done and what it would involve for you. Sam Chenery-Morris will go through the information sheet with you and answer any questions you have. This should take about 10 minutes. Talk to other mentors or students about the study if you wish. (Part 1 tells you the purpose of this study and what will happen to you if you take part. Part 2 gives you more detailed information about the conduct of the study). Ask if there is anything that is not clear.

Part 1

What is the purpose of this study?

The NMC decided that all midwifery practice should be graded, as this is the first time this university, and many others in the UK, have undertaken this process; I would like to explore how you, as students and mentors feel about it.

Why have I been invited?

Because you are a midwifery mentor or student midwife and involved in the grading process. I would like your thoughts and feelings on the grading process.

Do I have to take part?

It is up to you to decide to join the study. I will describe the study and go through this information sheet. If you agree to take part, I will then ask you to sign a consent form. You are free to withdraw at any time, without giving a reason.

What will happen to me if I take part?

Following the grading process, I would like to individually interview mentor volunteers and form a focus group with students. This means approximately one hour of your time for each session. I will come to a place convenient to you, probably a private room in the hospital or education centre. If we have routine tripartite meetings they will be used as a time for reflection for students, mentors and lecturers and myself, to examine the process of grading and interactions during the meeting.

Will there be expenses and payments?

There are no incentives or payments for undertaking this research.

What are the possible disadvantages and risks of taking part?

In the interviews I will be asking you about your feelings, feelings are complex and this may be hard for some people. If you would like support to discuss your feelings, outside this research project, you can be referred to or self-refer to student services. The student services team are committed to offering a free, confidential, impartial and experienced service, offering one to one advice and guidance.

What are the possible benefits of taking part?

The benefit of this research is that you may understand the grading process more, as a student and a mentor.

Will my taking part in the study be kept confidential?

Yes. We will follow ethical and legal practice and all information about you will be handled in confidence. All interview and focus group data will be confidential.

If the information in Part 1 has interested you and you are considering participation, please read the additional information in Part 2 before making any decision.

Part 2

If you have a concern about any aspect of this study, you should ask to speak to the researcher Sam Chenery-Morris who will do her best to answer your questions [01473 338644]. *If you remain unhappy and wish to complain formally, you can do this* [University research services 01603 591574].

Will my taking part in this study be kept confidential?

Data will be collected in person, by interviews or focus groups. This information will be audio recorded. It will be stored securely anonymously on a password secured computer. If you join the study, some parts of the data collected for the study will be looked at by authorised persons, such as my supervisor from UEA. They may also be looked at by authorised people to check that the study is being carried out correctly. All will have a duty of confidentiality to you as a research participant and we will do our best to meet this duty.

Who is funding this study?

No-one is funding this study; it is being undertaken by me as part of an academic process.

Who has reviewed this study?

All research in the NHS is looked at by an independent group of people, called a Research Ethics Committee, to protect your interests. This study has been reviewed and given favourable opinion by East of England Research Ethics Committee and each hospital research and development site.

Further information and contact details

For more information or to discuss this project please ring or e-mail
01473 338644 or s.chenery-morris@ucs.ac.uk

All study participants will be provided with a copy of the Information Sheet and Consent Form for their personal records. Your rights are straightforward, you have the right to participate or not, even if you participate you have the right to withdraw at any time. There will be no problem or come back if you choose to withdraw, participation or non-participation will not affect your continuing midwifery education. Ask any question if some part of the information is not clear to you or if you would like more information.

Appendix 3

Interview questions

Version 1; 10/H0310/45 for mentors

Written 4 October 2010
   Pilot study – Grading midwifery practice – Sam Chenery-Morris

1. What is your experience of being a mentor?
2. Have you previously graded midwifery practice?
3. Did the workshops and/or triennial review study days prepare you for grading students?
4. What is your experience of delivering feedback?
5. What are the strengths and limitations of this form of assessment?
6. Can you reflect on the assessment process?
7. How did you find the terminology used within the assessment tool? (Tool attached)
8. What else do you look for in a student when you assess them?
9. What do you think the student expects from the assessment process?
10. Any other comments.

Student group interview schedule Version 1; 10/H0310/45 for students

Written 4 October 2010
   Pilot study – Grading midwifery practice – Sam Chenery-Morris

1. What was your experience of the grading process?
2. How did you find the self-assessment of your practice element of the grade?
3. How did you find the mentors assessment of your practice?
4. What was your experience of the negotiation of the grade?
5. Were there differences between different mentors?
6. Were the assessments conducted in work time?
7. What was the environment of the assessment?
8. How did you find the terminology on the grading tool?

Any other points about grading?

Interview schedule for midwifery mentors, Version 2

Written July 2012

Grading pre-registration midwifery practice – Sam Chenery-Morris

1. What is your experience of being a mentor?
2. Have you previously graded midwifery practice?

3. There are four areas that are assessed within the grading process, how did you feel these are measured, and what do they mean to you?

Effective midwifery practice
Professional and ethical practice
Developing the individual midwife and others
Achieving quality care through evaluation and research

4. Did the workshops and/or triennial review study days prepare you for grading students?
5. What is your experience of delivering feedback?
6. Can you reflect on the a``ssessment process?
7. How did you find the terminology used within the assessment tool?
8. What else do you look for in a student when you assess them?
9. What do you think the student expects from the assessment process?
10. Does grading affect the relationships you develop with students?

Any other comments.

Student group interview schedule Version 2

Written July 2012

Grading pre-registration midwifery practice – Sam Chenery-Morris

1. What was your experience of the grading process?
2. There are four areas that are assessed within the grading process how did you feel these are measured, and what do they mean to you?

Effective midwifery practice
Professional and ethical practice
Developing the individual midwife and others
Achieving quality care through evaluation and research

3. How did you find the self-assessment of your practice element of the grade?
4. How did you find the mentors assessment of your practice?
5. What was your experience of the negotiation of the grade?
6. Were there differences between different mentors?

7. Where were the assessments conducted?
8. How did you find the terminology on the grading tool?
9. How does having your practice graded affect the relationships with your mentors?
10. Any other points about grading

Appendix 4

Participant consent sheet

Participant Identification Number for this study:
(Prefix S for student, M for mentor, and L for lecturer)

Sample consent form for pilot research study
Title of project: Evaluating grading midwifery practice
Name of researcher: Sam Chenery-Morris

Please tick to confirm

- I confirm that I have read and understand
  the information sheet dated..........................
  (version............) for the above study.

- I have had the opportunity to consider the
  information, ask questions and have had these
  answered satisfactorily.

- I understand that my participation is voluntary and
  that I am free to withdraw at any time, without giving
  any reason.

- I understand that relevant sections of any data
  collected during the study, may be looked at by
  responsible individuals from the university.

- I agree to take part in the above research study.

Name of Participant	Date	Signature

Name of Person taking consent (if different from researcher)	Date	Signature

Researcher	Date	Signature

When complete, one copy for participant: one copy for researcher file

Appendix 5
Ethical approval process

Table A5.1 Ethical approval process for pilot study

Date	Event	Outcome
October 2009	Started PhD	Pending
18 January 2010	Study University Ethics approval sought	Approved on 27 January 2010
27 January 2010	Sanderling University approval sought	Approved on 9 February 2010
9 February 2010	Registered with IRAS	Spent months filling in forms
9 August 2010	An English NHS LREC approval sought	Approved with conditions 19 September 2010 Conditions met November 2010 *Ref*: 10/H0310/45
January and February 2011	Local R and D approval needed	Site 1 approved February 2011 Site 2 not approved Site 3 approved January 2011

Table A5.2 Ethical clearance for the core phase of research

Date	Event	Date/outcome/ref
11 May 2012	Study University ethics approval sought	31 May 2012 Substantial revisions required 15 August 2012 approved
22 May 2012	Sanderling University ethics approval sought	9 September 2012 Approved after revisions
4 October 2012	IRAS approval sought	7 November 2012 IRAS signed 107146/381208/14/388
12 November 2012	Trust 2 approval sought	19 November 2012 approved 2012WCH005
15 November 2012	Trust 3 approval sought	19 November 2012 approved 2012/STU/04
9 November 2012	Trust 1 approval sought	22 April 2013 approved 2012/180

Appendix 6

Sanderling University approved grading tool (February 2009)

Appendix 6.1 The first grading tool

20–16	15–11	10–6	5–0	Mark awarded by		
				Student	Mentor	Agreed
Effective midwifery practice						
Excellent links made between knowledge and practice	Very good links made between knowledge and practice	Good links made between knowledge and practice	Limited links made between knowledge and practice			
Excellent understanding of the midwife's role	Very good understanding of the midwife's role	Good understanding of the midwife's role	Limited understanding of the midwife's role			
Consistently adapts language to ensure effective communication with women/families and the multi-disciplinary team	In most circumstances, adapts language appropriately. Occasional prompting required to ensure effective communication	In some circumstances able to adapt language appropriately. Needs prompting to ensure effective communication	Frequent prompting required to adapt language to ensure effective communication			
Excellent ability to assess the woman's needs and plan and participate in care appropriately	Very good ability to assess the woman's needs and plan and participate in care appropriately	Good ability to assess the woman's needs and plan and participate in care appropriately	Frequently requires support to assess the woman's needs and plan and participate in care appropriately			
Consistently demonstrates a women-centred approach to care based on partnership	On most occasions demonstrates a women-centred approach to care based on	Sometimes demonstrates a women-centred approach to care based on partnership	Requires ongoing support to demonstrate a women-centred approach to care based on partnership			
Dexterity demonstrated in skill development expected at level 1	Good skill development at level 1 though there is scope for refinement only in some areas	Skill development satisfactory for level-1 student	Some skills would benefit from further refinement for a level-1 student			

(Continued)

Comments

				Mark awarded by		
				Student	Mentor	Agreed
20–16	15–11	10–6	5–0			

Professional and ethical practice

20–16	15–11	10–6	5–0
Excellent ability to express personal feelings and identify learning from experience	Very good ability to express personal feelings and identify learning from experience	Good ability to express personal feelings and identify learning from experience	Support required to express feelings and identify learning from experience
Consistently displays an understanding of the concepts of professionalism	Frequently displays an understanding of the concepts of professionalism	On some occasions demonstrates an understanding of professionalism	Understanding of professionalism requires development in some areas
Consistently promotes ethical and non-discriminatory practices	Typically practices in accordance with ethical and non-discriminatory frameworks	Demonstrates an understanding of practice within ethical and non-discriminatory frameworks	Has understanding but demonstrates some hesitancy in attending to the individual rights, interests, beliefs and cultures of women
Consistently creates an environment of care to promote the health, safety and wellbeing of women	Frequently able to create an environment of care to promote the health, safety and wellbeing of women	Is able in some circumstances to creates an environment of care to promote the health, safety and wellbeing of women	Attempts to create an environment of care to promote the health, safety and wellbeing of women
Performs effectively within a multi-disciplinary team	Usually works well within a multi-disciplinary team	Aware of own contribution to multi-disciplinary team working	Some hesitancy of involvement within multi-disciplinary team
Demonstrates understanding and application of relevant legislation to practice commensurate with level 1	Understands relevant legislation to practice commensurate with level 1	Is able to identify some areas of relevant legislation commensurate with level 1	Needs support to identify legislative framework for practice commensurate with level 1

(Continued)

Comments

20–16	15–11	10–6	5–0	Mark awarded by		
				Student	Mentor	Agreed
Developing the individual midwife and others						
Proactively identifies and engages in learning opportunities within the practice environment for a level 1 student	Actively engaged in learning within the practice environment for a level 1 student	Seeks out learning opportunities with some encouragement for a level 1 student	Requires support to identify appropriate learning opportunities for a level 1 student			
Well-motivated within the practice arena	Shows enthusiasm in most practice areas	In some circumstances willing to engage in practice	Encouragement needed to engage in practice			
Consistently displays a mature attitude to receiving constructive criticism and adapts performance accordingly	Able to accept and use constructive criticism to improve performance	Accepts constructive criticism and makes efforts to improve performance	Requires support to interpret constructive criticism			
Consistently displays confidence appropriate for level 1	On most occasions shows confidence in practice appropriate for level 1	Confident in some situations appropriate for level 1	Level of confidence may adversely inhibit performance appropriate for level 1			
Consistently displays an empathetic approach to care	In most circumstances demonstrates an empathetic approach to care	In some circumstances demonstrates an empathetic approach to care	Needs help to demonstrate empathetic responses to care			
Makes good use of assertiveness skills to effectively care for women	Frequently uses assertiveness skills to effectively care for women	In some situations, demonstrates assertiveness skills to effectively care for women	Care for women would be enhanced if assertiveness skills were developed			

(Continued)

Comments

Achieving quality care through evaluation and research

20–16	15–11	10–6	5–0	Mark awarded by		
				Student	Mentor	Agreed
Explains methods used to monitor and evaluate care and performance	Identifies methods to monitor and evaluate care and performance	Needs encouragement to recognise methods used to monitor and evaluate care and performance	Limited ability to recognise methods used to monitor and evaluate care and performance			
Frequently draws on evidence to support care decisions	Sometimes draws on evidence to support care decisions	Needs some encouragement to consider evidence to practice	Limited recall on evidence to support practice			

Comments

Total of agreed marks awarded

Appendix 7

Sanderling University approved
grading tool (January 2011)

Table A7.1 Sanderling University approved grading tool (January 2011)

4	3	2	1	Mark awarded by		
				Student	Mentor	Agreed
Effective midwifery practice						
Excellent links made between knowledge and practice	Very good links made between knowledge and practice	Good links made between knowledge and practice	Limited links made between knowledge and practice			
Excellent understanding of the midwife's role	Very good understanding of the midwife's role	Good understanding of the midwife's role	Limited understanding of the midwife's role			
Consistently adapts language to ensure effective communication with women/families and the multi-disciplinary team	In most circumstances adapts language appropriately. Occasional prompting required to ensure effective communication	In some circumstances able to adapt language appropriately. Needs prompting to ensure effective communication	Frequent prompting required to adapt language to ensure effective communication			
Excellent ability to assess the woman's needs and plan and participate in care appropriately	Very good ability to assess the woman's needs and plan and participate in care appropriately	Good ability to assess the woman's needs and plan and participate in care appropriately	Frequently requires support to assess the woman's needs and plan and participate in care appropriately			
Consistently demonstrates a women-centred approach to care based on partnership	On most occasions demonstrates a women-centred approach to care based on	Sometimes demonstrates a women-centred approach to care based on partnership	Requires ongoing support to demonstrate a women-centred approach to care based on partnership			
Dexterity demonstrated in skill development expected at level 1	Good skill development at level 1 though there is scope for refinement only in some areas	Skill development satisfactory for level 1 student	Some skills would benefit from further refinement for a level 1 student			

(Continued)

Table A7.1 (Continued) Sanderling University approved grading tool (January 2011)

Comments	4	3	2	1	Mark awarded by		
					Student	Mentor	Agreed
Professional and ethical practice							
	Excellent ability to express personal feelings and identify learning from experience	Very good ability to express personal feelings and identify learning from experience	Good ability to express personal feelings and identify learning from experience	Support required to express feelings and identify learning from experience			
	Consistently displays an understanding of the concepts of professionalism	Frequently displays an understanding of the concepts of professionalism	On some occasions demonstrates an understanding of professionalism	Understanding of professionalism requires development in some areas			
	Consistently promotes ethical and non-discriminatory practices	Typically practices in accordance with ethical and non-discriminatory frameworks	Demonstrates an understanding of practice within ethical and non-discriminatory frameworks	Has understanding but demonstrates some hesitancy in attending to the individual rights, interests, beliefs and cultures of women			
	Consistently creates an environment of care to promote the health, safety and wellbeing of women	Frequently able to create an environment of care to promote the health, safety and wellbeing of women	Is able in some circumstances to creates an environment of care to promote the health, safety and wellbeing of women	Attempts to create an environment of care to promote the health, safety and wellbeing of women			

(Continued)

Table A7.1 (Continued) Sanderling University approved grading tool (January 2011)

4	3	2	1	Mark awarded by		
				Student	Mentor	Agreed
Performs effectively within a multi-disciplinary team	Usually works well within a multi-disciplinary team	Aware of own contribution to multi-disciplinary team working	Some hesitancy of involvement within multi-disciplinary team			
Demonstrates understanding and application of relevant legislation to practice commensurate with level 1	Understands relevant legislation to practice commensurate with level 1	Is able to identify some areas of relevant legislation commensurate with level 1	Needs support to identify legislative framework for practice commensurate with level 1			
Comments						
4	3	2	1			

Developing the individual midwife and others

4	3	2	1			
Proactively identifies and engages in learning opportunities within the practice environment for a level 1 student	Actively engaged in learning within the practice environment for a level 1 student	Seeks out learning opportunities with some encouragement for a level 1 student	Requires support to identify appropriate learning opportunities for a level 1 student			
Well-motivated within the practice arena	Shows enthusiasm in most practice areas	In some circumstances willing to engage in practice	Encouragement needed to engage in practice			

(Continued)

Table A7.1 (Continued) Sanderling University approved grading tool (January 2011)

Consistently displays a mature attitude to receiving constructive criticism and adapts performance accordingly	Able to accept and use constructive criticism to improve performance	Accepts constructive criticism and makes efforts to improve performance	Requires support to interpret constructive criticism
Consistently displays confidence appropriate for level 1	On most occasions shows confidence in practice appropriate for level 1	Confident in some situations appropriate for level 1	Level of confidence may adversely inhibit performance appropriate for level 1
Consistently displays an empathetic approach to care	In most circumstances demonstrates an empathetic approach to care	In some circumstances demonstrates an empathetic approach to care	Needs help to demonstrate empathetic responses to care
Makes good use of assertiveness skills to effectively care for women,	Frequently uses assertiveness skills to effectively care for women,	In some situations, demonstrates assertiveness skills to effectively care for women	Care for women would be enhanced if assertiveness skills were developed

(Continued)

Table A7.1 (Continued) Sanderling University approved grading tool (January 2011)

Comments

4	3	2	1	Mark awarded by		
				Student	Mentor	Agreed
Achieving quality care through evaluation and research						
Explains methods used to monitor and evaluate care and performance	Identifies methods to monitor and evaluate care and performance	Needs encouragement to recognise methods used to monitor and evaluate care and performance	Limited ability to recognise methods used to monitor and evaluate care and performance			
Frequently draws on evidence to support care decisions	Sometimes draws on evidence to support care decisions	Needs some encouragement to consider evidence to practice	Limited recall on evidence to support practice			

Comments

Total of agreed marks awarded

Appendix 8

Sanderling University approved
grading tool (May 2012)

Table A8.1 Sanderling University approved grading tool (May 2012)

	1–3	4	5	6	7–10	Mark awarded by		
						Student	Mentor	Agreed
Effective midwifery practice								
Application of midwifery knowledge to practice	Application of midwifery knowledge to practice limited	Applies some knowledge practice but needs to develop knowledge to enhance care	On most occasions applies appropriate knowledge and understanding to practice	Consistently able to apply appropriate links between knowledge and practice	Exceptionally able to apply rationale between knowledge and practice			
	Frequent prompting required to demonstrate the role of the midwife	Occasional prompting required to demonstrate the role of the midwife	On most occasions demonstrates the role of the midwife	Consistently able to demonstrate the role of the midwife	Exceptionally able to demonstrate the role of the midwife			
	Frequent prompting required to adapt language to ensure effective communication	In some circumstances able to adapt language appropriately. Needs prompting to ensure effective communication	In most circumstances adapts language appropriately. Occasional prompting required to ensure effective communication	Consistently adapts language to ensure effective communication with women/families and the multi-disciplinary team	Exceptional awareness and insight of communication skills with women, families and MDT			

(Continued)

Table A8.1 (Continued) Sanderling University approved grading tool (May 2012)

1–3	4	5	6	7–10	Mark awarded by		
					Student	Mentor	Agreed
Frequently requires support to assess, determine and plan programmes of care for women based on needs from preconception to the postnatal period	Demonstrates ability to assess, determine and plan programmes of care for women based on needs from preconception to the postnatal period with prompting	On most occasions demonstrates ability to assess, determine and plan programmes of care for women based on needs from preconception to the postnatal period without prompting	Consistently demonstrates ability to assess, determine and plan programmes of care for women based on needs from preconception to the postnatal period	Exceptional ability to assess, determine and plan programmes of care for women based on needs from preconception to the postnatal period			
Requires ongoing support to demonstrate a women-centred approach to care based on partnership which respects the individuality of women	Understands a women-centred approach to care based on partnership which respects the individuality of women although needs prompting to achieve	On most occasions demonstrates a women-centred approach to care based on partnership which respects the individuality of women	Consistently demonstrates a woman-centred approach to care based on partnership which respects the individuality of women	Demonstrates exceptional ability in woman-centred approach to care based on partnership which respects the individuality of women			

(Continued)

Table A8.1 (Continued) Sanderling University approved grading tool (May 2012)

1–3	4	5	6	7–10	Mark awarded by		
					Student	Mentor	Agreed
Limited opportunity for skill demonstration	Some skills would benefit from further refinement	Skill development satisfactory	Very good skill development	Dexterity demonstrated in skills			
Comments							
Professional and ethical practice							
Support required to engage in reflection on practice	Occasionally uses reflection to consider how care can be improved	Frequently uses *structured* reflection to consider how care can be improved	Uses structured reflection on practice to enhance care delivery without prompting	Exceptional ability to analyse care using reflection of own and wider influences			
Understanding of professionalism requires development in some areas	On some occasions needs reminding about aspects of professionalism	Frequently displays an understanding of the concepts of professionalism	Consistently displays an understanding of the concepts of professionalism	Professionalism maintained and demonstrated at all times, including role modelling for others			

(Continued)

Table A8.1 (Continued) Sanderling University approved grading tool (May 2012)

1–3	4	5	6	7–10	Mark awarded by		
					Student	Mentor	Agreed
Has understanding but demonstrates some hesitancy in attending to the individual rights, interests, beliefs and cultures of women	Demonstrates an understanding of practice within ethical and non-discriminatory frameworks	Typically practices in accordance with ethical and non-discriminatory frameworks	Consistently promotes ethical and non-discriminatory practices	Exceptional awareness and demonstration of ethics			
Unaware of environment of care to promote the health, safety and wellbeing of women	Is able in some circumstances to creates an environment of care to promote the health, safety and wellbeing of women	Frequently able to create an environment of care to promote the health, safety and wellbeing of women with prompting	Usually creates an environment of care to promote the health, safety and wellbeing of women on own initiative	Exceptional ability to create a caring environment for all women			
Some hesitancy of involvement with the team	Aware of own contribution to working within the team	Usually works well within the team	Consistently works well within the team	Excellent contribution within the team			

(Continued)

Table A8.1 (Continued) Sanderling University approved grading tool (May 2012)

1–3	4	5	6	7–10	Mark awarded by		
					Student	Mentor	Agreed
Needs support to identify legislative framework for practice	Is able to identify some areas of relevant legislation	Understands relevant legislation to practice	Demonstrates understanding and application of relevant legislation to practice	Exceptional knowledge and application of legislative frameworks to practice			

Comments

Developing the individual midwife and others

1–3	4	5	6	7–10			
Requires support to identify appropriate learning opportunities	Seeks out learning opportunities with some encouragement	Actively engaged in learning within the practice environment	Proactively identifies and engages in learning opportunities within the practice environment	Exceptional ability to enhance learning at every opportunity			
Encouragement needed to engage in practice	Willing to engage in practice	Shows enthusiasm in most practice areas	Well-motivated within the practice arena	Exceptionally well-motivated and engaged in all practice			

(Continued)

Table A8.1 (Continued) Sanderling University approved grading tool (May 2012)

1–3	4	5	6	7–10	Mark awarded by		
					Student	Mentor	Agreed
Requires support to interpret constructive criticism	Accepts constructive criticism and makes efforts to improve performance	Able to accept and use constructive criticism to improve performance	Consistently displays a mature attitude to receiving constructive criticism and adapts performance accordingly	Exceptionally able to reflect upon own practice performance to enhance care			
Level of confidence (high or low) may adversely inhibit performance	Appropriate confidence in some situations	On most occasions shows confidence in practice	Consistently displays confidence in practice	Performance exceptional confident to manage appropriate care in all circumstances			
Needs help to demonstrate empathetic responses to care	In some circumstances demonstrates an empathetic approach to care may need prompting	In most circumstances demonstrates an empathetic approach to care without prompting	Consistently displays an empathetic approach	Exceptional ability to empathise will all clients			
Care for women would be enhanced if assertiveness skills were developed	In some situations, demonstrates assertiveness skills to effectively care for women	Frequently uses assertiveness skills to effectively care for women,	Consistently utilises assertiveness skills to effectively care for women,	Exceptional ability to care and advocate for women			
Comments							

Table A8.1 (Continued) Sanderling University approved grading tool (May 2012)

1–3	4	5	6	7–10	Mark awarded by		
					Student	Mentor	Agreed
Achieving quality care through evaluation and research							
Needs encouragement to recognise processes such as audit and research that contribute to the monitoring and evaluation of care and performance	Able to identify methods to monitor and evaluate care and performance	Conversant with methods to monitor and evaluate care and performance, may need prompting to do so	Explains how monitoring can enhance care and performance and able to evaluate own contribution	Exceptional ability to audit own notes and apply research findings to care decisions			
Needs encouragement to consider evidence for practice	Sometimes draws on evidence to support care decisions	Frequently draws on evidence to support care decisions	Incorporates best available evidence into practice	Exceptional ability to seek out best available evidence			
Comments							
Total of agreed mark awarded							

Appendix 9

Example of open and axial codes

Table A.9.1 Examples of coding

Participants' words	Open coding	Axial coding
Sometimes if you've given a woman a piece of advice that you know is the right piece of advise ... if your mentor goes out of the room and she comes back in the room oh I'll say we were just discussing and re-iterate the whole conversation just to confirm	Communication with women	Visible pedagogy – student knew how to make her communication with women visible Strong classification of the advice as something important.
But its simple things like discussing a birth plan with a women, nine times out of ten the mentor's still outside and hasn't come in at this point and they won't sign you off because they haven't seen you discuss a birth plan	Communication with women	Invisible pedagogy student unable to make her communication with the woman visible to the mentor. In considering the birth plan simple it means the activity is weakly classified when it should be strong
I certainly feel I don't trust myself with anything that even the stuff that used to be my job and the example was that ... a lady rang up with bleeding in early pregnancy that was my job for five years and I said hang on I'll get the midwife	Confidence	Strong classification between previous role as a nurse and current role as a student midwife affected student's ability to give information she knew
I'm fine with my midwifery mentor watching me, no problem, but with others ... standing over you, I am not confident to say	Confidence	Difference between weak and strong framing affected student's confidence to practise and develop skills

Appendix 10

Teaching and learning literature search strategy

Search 1 student midwife or student midwives or midwifery
Search 2 midwi* mentor* or sign off mentor
Search 3 (1 or 2) (351 hits)
Search 4 UK or United Kingdom or Scotland or Wales or Northern Ireland or NI
Search 5 (3 and 4) (198 hits)
Search 6 research or study
Search 7 (5 and 6) (152)

Limiters peer reviewed and dates 2006–2017 (126)

When teaching and/or learning were added to the key words, there were no studies found from the UK, even though there were with the more generic search terms above.

Table A10.1 Decision re-inclusion, exclusion criteria

	Author name	Focus	Included	Rationale
1	Skirton	Newly qualified midwives	No	Not about students
2	Fisher	Grading practice	No	Not about teaching and learning
3	Moran	Value of role	Yes	
4	Afesth	Medical students	No	Not midwifery
5	Marshall	Erasmus scheme	No	No not specific
6	Finnerty	Practical coaching	Yes	
7	Baillie	Electronic health records	No	Not about teaching and learning
8	O'Brien	Preceptor role	No	Not about students
9	Longworth	Transfer of skills	Yes	
10	Chenery-Morris	Continuity of mentorship	No	My own work (therefore also implicit in thesis)
11	Haycock	Service users in assessment	No	Assessment focused
12	Collington	Link lecturer role	No	Useful for next chapter but not this one
13	Callwood	Multiple mini interviews	No	Not relevant
14	Young	Clinical decision making NQM	No	Not relevant
15	Fraser	MINT	Yes	Letting go and safe environment
16	Wilson	Perineal repair	No	About qualified midwives
17	Hughes	Guiding and controlling hands	Yes	
18	McIntyre	BFI competence thesis	No	Too specific
19	Power	Are students prepared for 21st century	No	Not research
20	Holland	FTP in Scotland	Yes	Basic clinical skills/good mentors and bad mentors
21	Rowan	Reflections on education programme	No	About PBL curricula
22	Young	Clinical decision making NQM	No	Full thesis
23	Rawnson	Case loading BUMP study	No	Not specific enough. Knowing the mentor
24	Walker	Sexual health knowledge	No	Interesting but too specific Role modelling, generic knowledge
25	Walker	Sexual health advice	No	repeat

(Continued)

Table A10.1 (Continued) Decision re-inclusion, exclusion criteria

	Author name	Focus	Included	Rationale
26	Marjan	Stress	No	Iranian study
27	Fry	case loading	No	Not research
28	Bradbury-Jones	Health visitors	No	
29	McIntyre	Taster course	No	
30	Armstrong	Mentors' influence on students	Yes	There are ways to challenge mentors
31	Weston	Storytelling	No	Not about learning in the clinical environment
32	Banks	Flying start	No	About preceptorship
33	Fisher	What do midwifery mentors need	Yes	
34	Lauder	FTP curricula	No	Data collected 2004–2005 and only 6% midwifery students
35	Baird	Autonomy	No	Not specific about teaching but interesting. Community and MLBU more autonomy, mentors' way
36	Duffy	Mentors in waiting	No	Not research
37	Finnerty, 2006	Empowering mentors	No	Although data collected 2000–2003 (although mentors say they learn from students).
38	Howard	Flying start	No	preceptorship
39	Dow	Simulation part 1	No	Not in clinical area
40	Duffy	Six Cs in mentorship	No	Not research
41	Wood	CPFs	No	No not research
42	Dow	Simulation part 3	No	Not in clinical practice
43	Magnusson	New roles	No	Not relevant
44	Weston	Significant birth stories	No	Not relevant
45	Gelling	Making the most	No	Not research
46	Nettleton	Mentorship schemes	Yes	Valuing mentorship, choosing to be a mentor and improving the system
47	Dougherty	Tripartite assessment	No	Not about teaching and learning
48	Darra	Assessing practice	No	Not research
49	Robson	Choosing midwifery	No	Not research
50	McIntosh	Six universities	Yes	

Table A10.2 Critique and summary of literature

Authors	Focus	Methodology	Participants	Findings	Weaknesses
Chenery-Morris	To explore the importance of continuity of mentorship for students	Case study	51 Students and 15 mentors	Continuity needed for relationship development, working with different levels of students aids or adds to the workload, different areas of work are more conducive to teaching and learning	My own work, therefore not used as a reference as implicit within the whole thesis
Kroll	To explore whether student midwives' experience of hospital based care enabled then to achieve proficiencies required to register as midwives	Case study – Mixed methods. In-depth semi structured interviews, focus groups and student diaries,	Student midwives (n=5) interviewed, midwives, nurses (n=9) postal questionnaire and maternity care assistants (n=7) focus group and 32 student diaries	Main finding culture of ward and mentorship. Student status as learners was not recognised – they were an extra pair of hands. different perception of students 18 months picked things up quickly. Long course needed more support. Quality of relationship crucial. Students left to work on their own in hospital setting. One to one community environment preferred.	Conducted from 2005 to 2007 in one trust

(Continued)

Table A10.2 (Continued) Critique and summary of literature

Authors	Focus	Methodology	Participants	Findings	Weaknesses
Moran and Banks, 2016	To explore the value in the role of mentors	Phenomenology with in-depth interviews	Five Scottish midwives	Eight themes. Mentors enjoy their role but some thought role should be a choice. They question whether students value their role, yet some said they did for continuity, feedback and planning. Iimited time to teach and support students. p.54 'from a little girl to a fantastic midwife' from a midwife not qualified that long. Responsible for whether they passed of failed- yet grading? Students kept mentors up to date.	Purposive sampling and no length of time stated for the in-depth interviews, especially as carried out at place of work
Rooke, 2014	Evaluation survey of the new standards	Three-phase survey	114 new sign off mentors, 37 mentorship students and 13 nursing and midwifery lecturers were positive about the introduction of the sign off mentors' role	Concerns were raised about the support available for sign off mentors. The requirement of one hour of protected time per final placement was considered hard to implement and workload issues.	Nurse centric

(Continued)

Table A10.2 (Continued) Critique and summary of literature

Authors	Focus	Methodology	Participants	Findings	Weaknesses
Fisher and Webb, 2008	To explore and prioritise the needs of midwifery mentors and investigate any relationship between these and duration of experience and/or level of qualification	Two stage cross sectional correlation study	Six mentors in an initial focus group then questionnaire to 82 mentors (57 returned completed)	15 needs initially identified by focus group, 3 further from literature. All 18 used in survey. Frequent shifts = continuity. Support needed, usually from the university and a break from students valued. Theoretical front loading was beneficial. Younger students with limited social skills seemed problematic and time in the community with these rather than 18 month students more difficult. Student attributes such as too little or too much life experience was beneficial and problematic. Mentors experience was valuable with or without additional qualifications. More experienced mentors needed a break more than less experienced staff.	Study took place prior to 2006 standard, howevertriangulation of findings good. Good response rate

(Continued)

Table A10.2 (Continued) Critique and summary of literature

Authors	Focus	Methodology	Participants	Findings	Weaknesses
Longworth, 2013	To examine the attitudes of students towards skills training and practice	Mixed methods	questionnaires sent to all 36 midwifery students in one university (33 returned) in wales and follow up interviews with six purposely selected students.	Most students had positive attitudes about skills in university and practice. Having a mentor that knows you is beneficial. Mentors observed (79%), went through the process (79%) and gave feedback (91%) although this was less for third years. Frustration between the university ideal and practice reality noted.	
Finnerty and Collington, 2013	To explore learning strategies used by mentors from the student perspective	Discourse analysis from audio diaries	14 student audio diaries	Learning strategies; role modelling, debriefing and fading were offered. (The extracts all seem positive and game playing is positive. But undermining not supportive in my study). What if scenarios seen in my study-scaffolding. Many mentor styles.	Data recorded 2003 (ten years to publication as secondary analysis but still powerful). Uses an underpinning framework. Mentor diaries were noted to be brief – use this to support my chapter (Continued)

Table A10.2 (Continued) Critique and summary of literature

Authors	Focus	Methodology	Participants	Findings	Weaknesses
McIntosh et al., 2013	Bigger project aim; to determine the value of midwifery teachers, therefore student attitudes to learning are important	Focus group part of a larger national survey. This paper is an illuminative case study.	120 senior students across six universities in 17 focus groups	Teach yourself midwifery (in theory and practice). Knowing it all, (separation of knowledge acquisition in university from confidence in practice) right way of doing things (as many midwives practise differently). and importance of physical skills. Not valuing soft skills and highly valuing hard skills. Research questionable. Means unresolved tensions between NMC, expectations of practice and university philosophy	Part of MINT, large study multi-site, therefore increased credibility, sample self-selected
Hughes and Fraser, 2011	To explore students' experience and view of mentoring and qualities of mentors	Qualitative longitudinal cohort study using focus groups	58 women on three-year course (two cohorts), four times focus groups over their course (three groups cohort 1 and six groups in cohort 2)	Relationships. Expectations, role models and mentorship experience. Continuity essential in the first year, less so in subsequent years as students look to mentors as role models. The community seems more receptive to students. The demand on hospital staff is a barrier to teaching.	The longitudinal element is good as students views change over time. Size of focus group seemed to vary across the span

(Continued)

Table A10.2 (Continued) Critique and summary of literature

Authors	Focus	Methodology	Participants	Findings	Weaknesses
Armstrong, 2010	To find out whether students were influenced by traditional practices of their clinical mentors	Questionnaires (survey) with Likert scales	145 student midwives (125 returned (86%), final year both programmes (3 year and 18 month) in five universities.	What students are taught in university does not equate to workplace realities. Practice was too busy and students lacked authority. maintaining the status quo and not challenging the mentor was a way to 'fit in'. If they did challenge there were ways to do this, it was harder with older more experienced staff and it could jeopardise their clinical assessment. Lecturers and mentors do not seem to communicate- gap. So students adopt the way of their mentor.	Literature review acknowledges strong hierarchical structure may suppress students. A pilot study tested the questionnaire. There were some contradictions in the findings which questions the validity of the survey
Fraser et al., 2013	To explore midwife teachers' contributions, rather than mentors but included students views	Three-phase study	Questionnaire, interviews, activity analysis, focus group and semi structured diary entries	Teachers could support skill acquisition (but this was not in clinical practice), understanding midwifery practice, having a role and offering support. Over protective mentors prevented student learning/ experience development. Practising skills in a safe area in skills lab.	Students may have felt they had to say teachers were good. The appendixes and detail in the larger NMC folders

(Continued)

Table A10.2 (Continued) Critique and summary of literature

Authors	Focus	Methodology	Participants	Findings	Weaknesses
				NQM thought they were competent but lacked confidence. MT should be involved in consistency of tripartite assessment.	
Holland et al., 2010	Five aims evaluate students FFP	Mixed method, three phases (only phase 2 reported in this paper)	Questionnaires, OSCE and curriculum evaluation, phase 2 semi structured interviews (some telephone) and focus groups	Fitness for practice (including clinical skills, safe and attitudes – low confidence), Preparation for practice (some students have no healthcare experience but taught basic skills in uni first – drug management not seen until later in course), being in practice (and fitting in – good and bad mentors) and practice and partnerships	Good distinction between knowing clinical skills and being competent and having confidence. A comprehensive study with multiple authors contributing to the analysis

Appendix 11
Negotiation of grades

The arrows in the appendix denote:

⇧ mentor raises students' grade,

⬜ appears as if grading undertaken together rather than independently as all student and mentor grades are the same,

⇩ mentor lowers student's self-assessed grade,

Lastly, missing data is stated.

Appendix lla Three-year student negotiated grades

	First year	Second year	Third year
sw/T1	S340/342 ⇧ agreed=347/400 87%	S70/75m ⇧ agreed= 74/80 93%	S70/80m ⇧ 80/80= 100%
sx/T1	S312/339⇧ agreed 331= 83%	S78/80⇧ agreed 79/80= 99%	S79/80m ⇧ agreed= 80/80 100%
Sa/T2	S70.5/76m ⇧ Agreed 76/80= 95%	S71/ no mentor grades only agreed 72/80 ⇧ = 90%	S158/200 no mentor grade agreed 176/200 ⇧ = 88%
Si/T2	16/2/11 S75/80m ⇧ agreed 77/80= 96%	S69/70m ⇧ agreed 71/80= 89%	(s172/171m)⇩ agreed =171.5/200 = 86%
Sb/T3	S62/62m ⬜ agreed 62/80= 77%	Only half grid stapled in student's PAD- 1= (**grade 80–89%**) ⇧	no student self-assessed grade 186/200= 93%
Sc/T3	S61/63m ⇧ agreed 63/80= 79%	S123/ 136m ⇧ agreed 136/200= 68%	s141/167m ⇧ agreed 167/200= 83%
Sj/ T3	S66/73m ⇧ agreed 73/80= 91%	S128/139m ⇧ agreed 140/200= 70%	S161/188m ⇧ agreed 188/200= 94%
Sm/T3	no data – student transferred in from another university	S134/140m ⇧ agreed 140/200= 70%	S128/130m⇧ Both mentors present. agreed 130/200= **65% capped at 40%**

(Continued)

	First year	Second year	Third year

Sn/T1	90%
	grading form not
	   included in PAD
		S138/137m⇩
		agreed 137/200=
		68.5%
			s184/187⇧
			agreed grade 187/200=
			**Final grade 93% capped
			   40%**

S19/T3/ G5	no data	s133/159m ⇧ agreed 158/200= **79%**	s147/178m ⇧ agreed 178/200= **89%**
S21/ T2/G	S60/72m ⇧ agreed 74/80= **93%**	S140/196m ⇧ agreed 193/200= **97.5%**	S183/178⇩ agreed 178/200= **89%**
S18/ T3/G	S67/72m ⇧ agreed 72/80= **90%**	S154/148m⇩ agreed 148/200= **74%**	S159/176m ⇧ agreed 176/200= **88%**
Sk/T2	S63/63m □ agreed 63/80= **79%** MLBU	80 % missing data	S196/196m □ agreed 196/200= **96%**

S35/T2/
  G8
	S142/142m □
	agreed 142/200=
	71%
		S148/134m⇩
		agreed 134/200=
		67% – CDS mentor did
		   not want to grade
		   student 4 months later.
			S174/180m ⇧
			agreed 180/200=
			90%

S39/T2/ G9	S72/67m⇩ agreed 68/80= **85%**	S167/155m⇩ agreed 155/200= **77.5%**	S163/180m ⇧ agreed 180/200= **90%**
S29/T2/ G7	S105/121m ⇧ agreed 119/200= **60%**	S127/146m ⇧ agreed 146/200= **73%**	S154/191m ⇧ agreed 190/200= **95%**
Sl/ T3	S 73/76m ⇧ Agreed 76/80= **95%**	S127/147m ⇧ agreed 147/200= **73.5%**	S177/180m ⇧ agreed 180/200= **90%**
S41/T3/ G9	S69/73m ⇧ agreed =73/80= **91%**	s173/174m ⇧ agreed 174/200= **87%**	S167/180m ⇧ agreed 180= **90%**
S31/T3/ G7	S68/78m ⇧ agreed 78= CDS **97.5%**	S90/101m ⇧ agreed 101/200= **50%**	S127/125m⇩ agreed 125/200= **62.5% capped at 40%**

analysis	Students:
	312–340/400=**78–
	  85%**
	60–75/80=**75–94%**
	105–142/200=**52–
	  71%**
	mentors
	339–342/400=**85%**
	63–80/80=**79–100%**
	121–142/200=**60–
	  71%**
		Students
		69–78/80=**86–96%**
		90–167/200=**45–84%**
		Mentor
		70–80/80=**88–100%**
		101–196/200=**50–98%**
			students
			70–79/80=**88–99%**
			127–196/200=**63–98%**
			mentors
			80/80=**100%**
			125–196/200=**62–98%**

Appendix 11b 78-week student negotiated grades

Student	First 6 months	End 78 weeks
Sd/T2	(319s/315m)⇩ agreed 316= 79%	(S315/332m) ⇧ agreed 332/400= 83%
Se/T3	(S292/282m)⇩ 282/400= 70%	(314s/314m) ▢ =**78.5%** capped at 40%
Sf/T1	(S294/314m) ⇧ agreed 313/400= 78%	(s314/358m) ⇧ agreed 354/400= **88.5%**
Sg/T1	(s330/342m) ⇧ agreed 341/400= 85%	(S341/362m) ⇧ agreed 360/400= 90%
Sh/T1	(S302/306m) ⇧ agreed 304/400= **78.5%**	(S349/349m) agreed 352/400⇧= 88%
Sv/T1	S266/356m ⇧ agreed 334/400 =**83.5%**	S75/76⇧ agreed= 76/80 95%
Su/T1	s246/330⇧ agreed 323/400= 81%	S77/75m⇩ agreed 75/80= 94%
analysis	Student self-assessed grades 246–330/400= 61–82% mentor grades 282–356/400=70–89% agreed grades **70–85%**	student self-assessed grades 314–352/400= **78–88%** and 75–77/80=**94–96%** mentor grades 314–362/400=**78–90%** and 75–76/80=**94–95%** agreed grades **78–95%**

Appendix 12

RAG rating from student PAD long placement feedback

Table A12.1 RAG rating for three-year student midwives' long placement feedback

Student	Year 1	Year 2	Year 3	Total long placements
Sa/T2	CDS (red) Community, (red) community, (red) CDS	CDS, (red) Community	MLBU (amber), Ward (amber), CDS, Community, MLBU	11
Sb/T3	CDS (amber) Community, CDS, (amber) Community	All short placements	CDS (amber) Ward (red) CDS (red) Community (amber)	8
Sc/T3	Community CDS (red) Community CDS	CDS	CDS (amber) Community CDS (red)	8
Si/T2	CDS (red) Community CDS (red) Community (amber)	Community CDS (red)	CDS (red) Ward (amber) MLBU (amber) CDS (red)	10
Sj/T3	Community (amber) CDS Community (amber) CDS (red)	CDS	Ward CDS (amber) Community (red) CDS (red)	9
Sk/T2	CDS Community (amber) MLBU (amber)	MLBU (amber)	CDS (amber) Community Ward MLBU CDS (red)	9

(Continued)

Table A12.1 (Continued) RAG rating for three-year student midwives' long placement feedback

Student	Year 1	Year 2	Year 3	Total long placements
Sl/T3	CDS Community Community CDS (red)	CDS Ward	Ward MLBU Community (red) CDS	10
Sm/T3	No data	All short placements	CDS Ward (red) CDS (red) Community	4
Sn/T1	Community (amber) Community (red) CDS (amber)	Community (amber) CDS	Ward (red) CDS (red) Community MLBU CDS (red)	10
S19/T3/G5	No data	All short placements	CDS (red) Ward (red) CDS (amber) Community (amber)	4
S35/T2/G8	Community CDS (amber) Community CDS (amber)	CDS	CDS Ward MLBU (amber) Community CDS	10
S29/T2/G7	Community CDS Community	CDS CDS (amber)	Ward CDS Community MLBU	9
S39/T2/G8	Community CDS Community	CDS (amber)	Community Ward MLBU Community CDS	9
S21/T2/G5	Community (red) CDS (amber) Community (amber) CDS	CDS	Ward (amber) CDS (red) CDS (red) Community MLBU	10
S18/T3/G5	Community MLBU (amber) CDS (amber) Community	CDS (amber)	Ward (amber) CDS Community (red) CDS (amber)	9
S41/T3/G9	Community CDS (amber)	CDS (amber) Community	Community CDS MLBU Ward (amber) Community	9

(*Continued*)

Table A12.1 (Continued) RAG rating for three-year student midwives' long placement feedback

Student	Year 1	Year 2	Year 3	Total long placements
S31/T3/G7	Community CDS (red) Community (red) CDS (red)	All short placements	CDS (red) MLBU (red) Community (amber)	7
S2/T1/G1	Community (red) Community (amber) MLBU	CDS (red) Community	Ward (red) Community CDS (red) Community	9
S4/T1/G1	Community (amber) CDS (red) Community (red)	Community (red) CDS (amber)	CDS (amber) Ward (amber) CDS Community MLBU (amber)	10
Totals	60	23	82	165

Table A12.2 RAG rating of 78-week student evaluations

Student	1st 6 months	Last year	Total long placements
Sd/T2	Community CDS (amber) Ward (red)	Community CDS CDS	6
Se/T2	Community CDS (red) Ward (amber)	CDS (amber) Community (amber) CDS Ward	7
Sf/T1	CDS (amber) Ward (amber) Community	CDS Community CDS (amber) MLBU	7
Sg/T1	Ward CDS (red) Community	Community (red) CDS (amber) MLBU (amber)	6
Sh/T1	Ward (red) CDS Community	CDS (red) Community (amber) CDS (red) MLBU (red)	7
Su/T1	Ward CDS (red) Community	CDS MLBU Ward (red) Community	7
Sv/T1	CDS (amber) Ward Community	Community CDS CDS MLBU	7
Total	21	26	47

Index

Page numbers in 'bold' refer to tables; page numbers in 'italics' refer to figures.

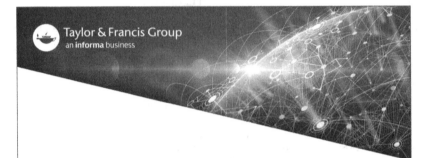

Printed in the United States
By Bookmasters